	DATE DUE	
APR 1 2 '95		

Here Tomorrow

JANET K. BELSKY

Here Tomorrow

Making the Most of
Life after Fifty

The Johns Hopkins University Press

BALTIMORE AND LONDON

© 1988 The Johns Hopkins University Press
All rights reserved
Printed in the United States of America

Originally published, 1988
Second printing, 1988

The Johns Hopkins University Press, 701 West 40th Street,
Baltimore, Maryland 21211
The Johns Hopkins Press Ltd., London

The paper used in this publication meets the minimum requirements of
American National Standard for Information Sciences—Permanence of
Paper for Printed Library Materials, ANSI Z39.48-1984.

Excerpts from chapter 4 are from *Love, Sex, and Aging: A Consumers
Union Report* by Edward M. Brecher and The Editors of Consumer
Reports Books. Copyright © 1984 by Consumers Union of United States,
Inc. By Permission of Little, Brown and Company.

All figures are from *Aging in America: Trends and Projects*, 1985–86 ed.,
published by the U.S. Senate Special Committee on Aging, Washington,
D.C., with the exception of Figure 1, which is from the *Chartbook on
Aging in America*, published by the National Council on the Aging,
Washington, D.C., 1981.

Library of Congress Cataloging-in-Publication Data

Belsky, Janet, 1947–
Here tomorrow: making the most of life after fifty/
Janet K. Belsky
p. cm.   Bibliography: p.   Includes index.
ISBN 0-8018-3718-9 (alk. paper)
1. Aged—United States.   2. Aging—United States.   3. Self-
actualization (Psychology)   I. Title.
HQ1064.U5B36   1988   88-45418
305.2'6'0973—dc19   CIP

C O N T E N T S

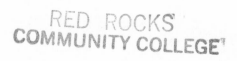

ACKNOWLEDGMENTS

This book would never have been published without the support of my agent, Maxine Groffsky, who steadfastly believed in my work, promptly read and reread the manuscript, and skillfully acted as my advocate through three changes of editors and three years of writing and rewriting. I also want to thank Alice Bennett, Therese Boyd, Nancy Essig, and especially Wendy Harris, my accomplished, reliable editor at Johns Hopkins University Press, for believing in this book and guiding me through the final stages. I am indebted to the many people I interviewed for enriching the following pages and to the experts in various aspects of aging who took time from their busy schedules to read and comment on the accuracy of specific chapters. And for giving me the confidence to begin and the stamina to persevere during the difficult times, I thank David, who made me a writer and has given me a happy life.

INTRODUCTION

Within the past few decades there has been an explosion of research on aging. Psychologists know how growing older affects memory, personality, our relationships, and the ways we view the world. They have information on everything from how grandparents feel and behave, to the emotional phases people go through after retiring, to how moving to a retirement community affects us mentally and physically. As a college teacher, psychologist, and textbook writer, I have spent years explaining and interpreting the gerontological research to students. I decided to write this book to help make this immensely relevant information available to everyone.

Here Tomorrow is for anyone interested in the latest research on growing older. It is also a very practical book, offering concrete suggestions for dealing with problems as different as getting along with your sixty-year-old daughter (or ninety-year-old mother-in-law), handling the first year of widowhood, and knowing where to go if you are afraid your father may have Alzheimer's disease. Until now, genuinely scientific information on most topics relevant to the second half of adult life has not been available in a single place. This book offers the first one-stop, psychologically oriented synopsis of what gerontologists know.

In each of the following ten chapters, I will be summarizing the latest research and offering step-by-step strategies for using this knowledge to build a more fulfilling life. I also will be providing information about where to go: the many programs, services, and opportunities now available to Americans in their fifties and beyond.

The first three chapters are about how growing older changes us. Chapter 1, "The Body," deals with physical aging. What underlies physical aging? What are the normal physical changes that occur in some important systems of our body during the second half of life? How can we differentiate normal aging from a disease that needs treatment, keep normal aging from shading into disability, and stick to the good health habits that the studies clearly show can help prevent chronic disease?

In chapter 2, "The Mind," I describe the latest research on intelligence and memory. What intellectual skills improve and what functions decline as we age? What is memory, and exactly how does it change in the second half of life? In the final sections of this chapter, I offer practical suggestions for enhancing thinking and improving memory.

Chapter 3 is about the emotional side of life—personality. Do people really change as the years pass? Is it true that age brings maturity? Who changes for the better, and who changes for the worse? How can you recognize whether you are depressed? This chapter ends with a variety of suggestions for enriching your life.

The next two chapters are about relationships. In chapter 4 I discuss long-lasting marriages and review the fascinating studies of newlyweds and new lovers over age fifty. Then I turn to sexuality. Which sexual changes are normal and which are not? How can you adapt your lovemaking to aging or deal with that abnormal change, impotence? How does menopause or a heart attack affect sexual functioning? Chapter 5 explores family relationships—adult children and elderly parents, the latest research on grandparenthood.

Chapters 6, 7, and 8 deal with life changes: "Retirement" (chap. 6), "Widowhood" (chap. 7), and "Living Arrangements and Changing Residence" (chap. 8). In chapter 6 I describe what motivates people to leave work early or to continue working beyond age sixty-five. How common is age discrimination in the workplace? How does retirement affect people economically, physically, and emotionally? Do retirees go through predictable stages in adjusting? What can you do to plan a fulfilling retired life?

Chapter 7, "Widowhood," explores the research on how people adjust emotionally to this common tragedy of middle and later life. What are the symptoms of bereavement? What does "recovering from mourning" mean? What constitutes normal versus pathological grief? Is losing a spouse more difficult for men than for women? At the end of this chapter I offer advice for married people, friends and relatives of widows and widowers, and widowed people themselves.

Chapter 8 describes the psychological research on moving and explores new housing alternatives for older people. How does changing residence affect us emotionally and physically? What are retirement communities like? What are the pluses and minuses of continuing-care retirement communities? What choices are open to the vast majority of older people who don't want to move?

The final two chapters are about illness. In chapter 9, "Dementia," I give a clear explanation of "senility," describing its symptoms, the illnesses that cause it, how diagnoses are made, and how close we are to cures. This chapter also covers research on how this devastating set of illnesses affects families, and it provides practical suggestions on how to cope.

Chapter 10, "Disability and Health Care," offers advice on dealing with disabling illness and finding appropriate medical care. What should you look for in choosing a doctor? What are the community alternatives to nursing homes? If a relative does need nursing-home care, how can you select the right place, prepare the person for the trauma of the move, and ensure that your family member gets good care as a resident?

The book ends with an Epilogue offering information on second careers after retirement, volunteer work, furthering your education, and pursuing an interest in the arts.

Here Tomorrow is written mainly for the intelligent older person (some sections are for family members dealing with an older relative). But because it should appeal to professionals too, I have included extensive citations for the studies I discuss. Do not be distracted by the notes scattered throughout each chapter; they are mainly for the convenience of professional readers. And understand that this book does not have to be read cover to cover. It is designed to be kept as a reference and consulted when a particular topic becomes a compelling concern.

The information in the following chapters is factual, not inspirational. Yet many of the scientific facts are as uplifting as a sermon would be. For instance, today "old age" starts closer to eighty-five than sixty-five; the latest research suggests that age does bring emotional maturity; older people are surprisingly resilient, even when confronting the worst tragedies (such as widowhood) growing old can bring. In fact, many people find that the decades after fifty, far from being an era of illness and unhappiness, are the most deeply satisfying time of life. I hope this book will encourage you and your loved ones to make these years of full maturity and unparalleled freedom the pinnacle they deserve to be.

PART

I

THE SELF

CHAPTER

1

THE BODY

In the past few years, since my seventy-fifth birthday, I have had to take my physical self in hand. It's not what I see in the mirror; the angular features, the bony face, the protruding eyes I always saw as so unattractive are still there, but their meaning has changed. What used to be strange looking has been transformed into what is so happily visible—a remarkable-looking older man! My body still looks hard and well proportioned. It was always much better than average. Now, in a bathing suit among people my age, it ranks almost off the scale. I love parading around half-naked and getting the many compliments I do about the way aging has treated the external me. To keep that envy coming, I am careful about exercising and what I eat. But I feel what has happened inside.

My checkups are perfect. My heart, which (like most men) I have been afraid would do me in, seems fine. Except for high blood pressure, my medical test results are all within normal limits. No one can believe how healthy I am. But I am not the same man I used to be.

I have trouble with the extremes of life. I am comfortable driving during the day, but not at night. What used to be darkness has become pitch black. What had been bright headlights are blinding. I dread facing an approaching car. And more than my sight has made driving hard. The last time I accelerated to get on the highway, it seemed as if I was moving underwater. By the time I swung my eyes around and got my foot on the gas pedal, the car far behind me was almost there, and I was inches from death.

I am less in control of my body at other times. I loved to

gorge myself. Now I have to eat slowly; spicy food makes me sick. I am more aware of the other end of my plumbing. Sometimes I sit on the toilet for hours. Hearing is more difficult at parties and restaurants.

From this description you would think that old age has emerged the conqueror, that I have given myself over to my limitations. Not so! It has a powerful adversary in me!

With ingenuity, I am able to live almost as full a life as ever. The key is to change the externals of my enjoyment to preserve the essential pleasures of life. Knowing what I cannot do, I orchestrate the outer scene to fit the new, internally different me. I don't go to restaurants. I have people come to the house. I have remodeled it to maximize the hearing I do have. I still go out at night, but I carry a flashlight; I take the bus. My love of people emerges unscathed. So does my love of food. I now relish each bite. Those five-minute dinners have become a half-hour to relax.

It's also surprising how much a regular swim helps with the slowing down. Now that I feel elderly, I—who have always seen the glass as half full—appreciate life's gifts more than ever. Pleasures like spending an evening with friends come harder, so the real value of friendship shines through. I love a good fight. Mind against matter; giving that enemy old age a run for its money. Sometimes I emerge victorious!

This man is fighting his own war against aging. How well are we doing as a nation? During this century, how far have we come at fighting aging and death?

As these simple statistics show, remarkably far: An American baby born in 1900 could expect to live to age forty-eight. His great-grandchildren, born in 1984, can expect to live an extra quarter-century, to age seventy-four. During these brief eight decades, life expectancy has increased more than a generation.

But our pace is slowing. As figure 1 shows, the upward curve of life expectancy is leveling off. As we push life expectancy upward, we approach a barrier we cannot go beyond, the biologically determined maximum limit of human life. This genetically fixed age limit, beyond which we are all programmed to die, is about age 110. And in the second half of our *possible*

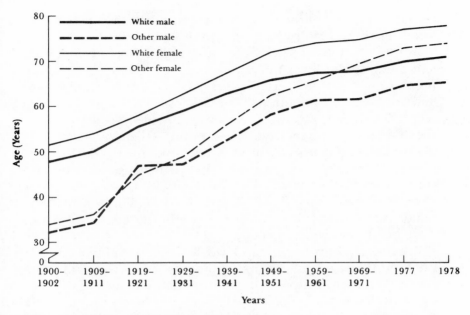

Figure 1   Life expectancy at birth, 1900-1978

life span, we encounter a set of illnesses related to the aging process—chronic diseases.

Our Enemy as We Age: Chronic Disease

There are two basic types of illnesses: infectious and chronic diseases. Infectious diseases are caused by microorganisms, invaders from outside the body. Examples are the flu, pneumonia, the common cold. Infectious diseases tend to come on quickly, lay us low for a few days or weeks, and usually go away without causing permanent harm. In contrast, internal breakdown is characteristic of chronic diseases. Although a few chronic illnesses are caused by known viruses, most have no identifiable outside cause. They usually involve permanent pathological changes produced by the body itself. They tend to develop slowly, get progressively worse, and have no cure. Though younger people too suffer from them, chronic diseases most often develop in middle and later life. They are related to the deterioration of the body that occurs as we age—rare in our twenties, more and more common in later years.

In 1900 the top causes of death in America were tuberculosis and pneumonia, both infectious diseases. Dramatic medical breakthroughs in the early decades of this century made these and other serious infectious illnesses less of a threat. Vaccines were developed; antibiotics became widespread. Because these diseases are relatively age blind, killing at three and eighty-three, these breakthroughs allowed most people to survive past youth. Life expectancy shot up because we now routinely live to the second half of the life span to encounter chronic diseases (see fig. 2). By the end of World War II our major killers had changed: our nation's top causes of death were heart disease and cancer.

Because the chronic diseases we develop in middle and later life tend to arise from the aging process itself, they are more difficult to fight. But we are limiting their advance. Our progress shines out not by looking at life expectancy at birth but by considering the additional years we can expect to live once we reach age sixty-five. In 1960 a man turning sixty-five could expect to live to seventy-seven, a woman to eighty-one. Men and women having sixty-fifth birthdays in 1983 could expect to live about three years longer, to ages 79.5 and 84.

The chances of living to our eighties and nineties rise with each passing year. People over eighty-five are the fastest-growing part of the population. The numbers of our oldest old are increasing at an astonishing rate.

Are these gains a Faustian bargain, time tacked on to the end of our life span at the price of suffering longer with chronic diseases? A study published by gerontologist Erdman Palmore in 1986 answers a resounding no.[1] Palmore compared surveys conducted by the National Center for Health Statistics from 1960 to 1980. In these government surveys, taken every few years, thousands of Americans are asked about their illnesses, their health problems, their physical limitations. When this Duke University researcher looked at health problems among people over sixty-five, he found less infirmity in 1980 than in 1970, less disability in 1970 than in 1960. Rather than severe physical problems multiplying as the ranks of the very old have increased, older people as a group are in better and better health.

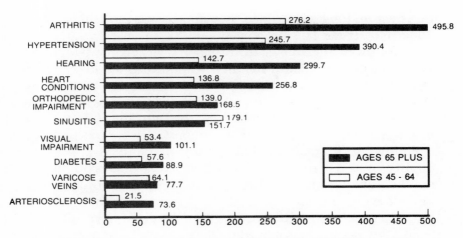

Figure 2   Top ten chronic conditions among the elderly, 1982 (rates per 1,000 persons)

One reason is that we now reach sixty-five healthier than ever. Many of us are physically middle-aged at the time society defines us as senior citizens (in our sixties) because we have eaten better, lived and worked in more healthful environments, and had better medical care all along. The revolution in what is happening *after* sixty-five has had an impact too. Within the past two decades the silver-haired marathon runner has overtaken the image of the passive older person staring into the sunset as our national old-age ideal. People in their sixties, seventies, and eighties are exhorted to stay young and vigorous. The sermons are not just wishful prayer. We now have proof that good health practices followed after middle age do dramatically extend life.

At the 1986 meeting of the American Psychological Association, George Kaplan reported on a large-scale life-expectancy study that has been going on since 1965 in Alameda County, California.[2] Nine thousand residents of the county have been followed over the years to determine the effect that habits such as not smoking, controlling weight, and exercising regularly have on mortality. It had been thought that following these life-extending practices after middle age would have little effect on longevity, since the damage was probably already done. Not true! The life expectancy of the men who at age sixty followed all three healthful habits was eighty-two, seven years longer than that of the men who followed none. Even at age eighty there was a significant difference in longevity between the two groups—1.5 years. And if a person changed any of these risk factors *after* age sixty, the mortality odds shifted too. In fact, it was never too late to partially reverse damage.

Following these simple habits also markedly affected life's quality, not just its length. The sixty-year-olds who did not smoke, exercised, and kept their weight within normal bounds were not only more likely to survive to their eighties but also much more likely to be *healthy* eighty-year-olds.

So there is no magic age when we can smoke or overdose on chocolates secure in the knowledge that it is too late anyway. But the results of this study are liberating in a more fundamental way. In later life people have more sway over their physical fate than was ever thought possible.

Even eighty is losing its once-sure standing as an old-age entry point. In a recent survey, one-fourth of the men and one-fifth of the women over eighty said they did not feel old. They were not assaulted by serious health problems or doubled over by aches and pains. One respondent in this large national survey puzzled: "The calendar tells me I'm old, but I still feel middle aged."[3]

What about being even older, over eighty-five? Surely the vast majority of people at this advanced age are beset by those physical problems that make us ask, "But at what price?" When University of Miami demographer Charles Longino looked at the incidence of severe physical disabilities among the 2,240,065 Americans over age eighty-five in the 1980 census, he found some startling facts. Only 47.8 percent had health problems that severely limited their ability to function. Most were living independently, not with their children or in a nursing home. Even in advanced old age the odds are less than fifty-fifty of having the infirmities that make life more a burden than a gift.[4]

The reason these odds seem so improbably low is that the older people who *are* severely disabled are the ones who stand out. Strolling through the city, our eye is drawn to the eighty-five-year-old in a wheelchair. We are oblivious to his contemporary vigorously striding by because he blends in with everyone else. Like any disaster, infirmity captures our attention. We then apply it to everyone because it fits our notions of what the late eighties and nineties have to be like.

We Age Differently

Not only is it wrong to label all eighty-five-year-olds "infirm," it is also untrue that at fifty everyone is physically middle-aged. Because of poor genetics, an unhealthful life-style, or bad luck, some fifty-year-olds function as if they were eighty; even some forty-year-olds are physically old.

In our nation's most comprehensive study of physical aging, now going on at the National Institute on Aging laboratories in Baltimore, researchers are finding that as we grow older making physical generalizations based on chronological age becomes harder and harder.[5] As the years advance, we become increasingly different from our contemporaries in our health and physical capacities. Ironically, by our sixties, the very time of life when we are lumped together as "senior citizens," the variations in aging rates are so striking that assigning any label seems particularly wrong.

Being older is usually an abstraction; there are so few changes in the way I feel. My back has begun to bother me more, and I can't see as easily or as well. But my energy level was always high, and I still can get around just as well. With some extra effort I still look almost the same as twenty years ago. It's more trouble to keep the weight off and cover that deep line I noticed last year. But I am mistaken for closer to forty than my real age, sixty-eight.

I am aware of approaching seventy only when I look at friends. There are such shocking differences in how old we look, and this is the time of life when our ranks begin to thin. Last week we went out to dinner with a couple, and the woman—a few years younger than me—had had a stroke and was in a wheelchair. I thought she looked more like my mother. I wondered at my incredible good luck.

How old or young we look is a fascinating clue to our rate of aging. In the National Institute on Aging study, researchers find that people who look middle-aged at seventy are more likely to be aging slowly internally too. But they caution that there is little relation between how we appear and how we function, mainly because making generalizations such as "he is young (or old) for his age" is so difficult. Our body systems themselves age at different rates. At sixty our heart may be physiologically eighty while our kidneys are like those of a thirty-year-old.

In other words, aging advances very differently—both between people and within ourselves. However, there are some generalizations we can make: the process itself occurs in definite ways. What exactly are these ways? This landmark National Institute on Aging study—called the Baltimore Longitudinal Study of Aging—offers answers to this question too.

Charting Normal Aging

As recently as a few decades ago, scientists knew little about how people normally change physically as they get older. Medical tests and treatments were based on what was right for a young adult, though most of us are diagnosed and treated medically in middle and later life. Doctors knew the bodies of their older patients were different, but they had to use laboratory standards based on young people for testing and treating seventy-year-olds. The dosages of drugs they gave often seemed too high for their older patients; they had been calibrated on volunteers in their twenties and thirties, when our body is in peak physical shape.

The Baltimore Longitudinal Study of Aging was begun in 1959 to shed light on how we change physiologically as we age. A group of reasonably healthy community-dwelling adults ranging from the teens to the late nineties was recruited. So far, about 650 men and 350 women have volunteered. People who enter the study are asked to make a lifelong commitment. Depending on their age, they return either every year or every two years to spend several days at the Gerontology Research Center in Baltimore answering questions about their health and undergoing tests. At each visit a comprehensive medical history is taken. Volunteers are thoroughly examined physically. Hundreds of capacities are measured, from grip strength to the amount of body fat to how fast the person can respond to a signal. Participants in the study are also given tests of memory and problem solving. Their personalities and mental health are plumbed.

Why don't the National Institute on Aging researchers simply compare how people of different ages function on these tests rather than requiring volunteers to make an ongoing commitment of this magnitude? The reason is that their approach—while demanding—provides a much more accurate picture of how aging occurs. Because each generation is arriving at eighty healthier, comparing today's forty-year-olds with today's eighty-year-olds would give a grossly inflated picture of the toll the years take. We are much safer if we measure that toll as it actually occurs—in flesh-and-blood human beings.

The Baltimore study has changed medical practice by giving doctors true age norms for interpreting laboratory tests. For instance, it has shown that the blood sugar level used for diagnosing diabetes, while adequate for a younger person, is too low to apply to a person past midlife. The body adjusts to a normal decrease in our ability to metabolize sugar as we get older, and the same laboratory reading that means a person in his twenties is diabetic may not signify diabetic symptoms in someone of sixty-five. Blood pressure that would upset us in a twenty-year-old may even be optimal for health in our seventies. We naturally need a higher blood pressure to circulate blood through arteries that are seventy years old. And the study is teaching doctors to tread more cautiously when they prescribe medicines. Lower dosages are often needed in later life.

THE DIFFERENT PATTERNS OF AGING

The landmark investigation at the National Institute on Aging is revealing that rather than just "declining," we change in several discrete ways as the years advance. One aging pattern is not to change at all. Although this happens with some bodily functions, the primary examples are not in the physical arena but in the mental one. As we will see in the next two chapters, personality and, in some important respects, intelligence tend to stay stable at least until advanced old age.

In another common pattern loss does occur, but only when a person develops an age-related illness. For instance, whereas it had been thought that in his middle and later years a man's body generally produces less and less testosterone (the male sex hormone), the Baltimore researchers found declining testosterone levels only in older subjects who were physically ill.

In yet a third pattern a loss does universally occur, but our body compensates physiologically for the change so we can function almost as well as ever. A fascinating example is the brain. As the years pass, individual brain cells are constantly lost; but the cells that remain make up for this erosion by becoming more robust. They grow new branches and new interconnections to compensate, and our thinking is preserved.

So the traditional view of aging as irreversible loss is wrong. A good deal of what seemed to be deterioration caused by being sixty or seventy turns out to be caused by being an *ill* sixty- or seventy-year-old. Many changes once seen as inevitable are potentially more reversible than anyone ever thought. And even when the years themselves take a physical toll, our bodies are surprisingly resilient. We have the capacity to grow and adapt in some surprising areas (such as the brain) where scientists never believed growth could occur after maturity.

HOW NORMAL AGING
AFFECTS US

The losses that do take place affect how we function in a special way. As we get older our ability to perform at top physical capacity gradually declines. Luckily, each of our body systems has a capacity greater than needed for normal living, so what is happening is noticeable only if we must stretch ourselves to our physical limit or if the changes have progressed so far that they interfere with daily life.

For example, to an athlete the small physical losses that happen early on are painfully apparent. At thirty-five he curses his "age" for making him lose the race to a younger man. Most of us are aware of these internal changes only years later. In our forties it is harder to play a strenuous game of tennis; we don't bounce back as fast from surgery. The physiological losses aging causes become a daily fact of life only when they have progressed even further. In our seventies we may have to take our bodies into account in planning our day. Normal aging has finally permeated ordinary life.

We instinctively understand what is happening when at about age fifty we start avoiding the extremes of life: "Should I run for that bus a block ahead?" "Should I go out in that hundred-degree heat?" "Maybe I should stay in bed, even if it is just a cold." Intuitively, we know. The words "everything in moderation" have begun to ring personally true.

But understanding that growing older means living a more temperate life does not mean taking to a wheelchair in the name of moderation. The old saying "the less we do, the less we can do" is just as valid a phrase to live by. When we act as if we cannot do something, although we can, eventually that physical function really does go. In fact, the best way to react to physical aging is to view what is happening as a challenge— a chance to use creativity to rearrange your life so that what has occurred does not keep you from living fully.

Let's first look briefly at how aging affects the cardiovascular and respiratory systems (where the words "the less we do, the less we can do" are especially true), then explore how we might apply this environmental engineering to three other important body systems—vision, hearing, and digestion. What specific changes can we expect as we grow older? How can we arrange our lives to minimize the effect of these minor losses?[6]

Because we all differ physically, the changes I describe below may be either more or less pronounced for you, depending on your unique rate of aging. And compensating totally on your own makes sense only when dealing with normal aging, not with disease. Since only a doctor can judge what is indeed normal, take the conservative course. Visit your physician when you notice *any* physical problem or change. Finally, if you do have a disability, turn to chapter 10; it offers information on how to deal with physical problems that limit life in a major way.

Specific Changes with Aging

CARDIOVASCULAR AND RESPIRATORY SYSTEMS

Our hearts and lungs work together to perform the vital function of making available the oxygen-rich blood that our cells need. The heart must pump blood continuously and at an adequate rate to get blood to our tissues. Our bellowslike lungs must fill and empty well enough to cleanse blood of the waste product of metabolism, carbon dioxide, and replenish the needed oxygen. As we grow older both these jobs are gradually performed less efficiently, and this becomes most apparent (and most serious) when we are pushing our bodies to the limit—when we exert ourselves physically.

There is a reduction in what is called "cardiac output." Our maximum heart rate during exercise does not get as high, and the volume of blood our heart can deliver per beat declines. The net effect is that our heart cannot circulate as much blood as quickly. This causes a decline in "maximum oxygen consumption," the peak amount of oxygen that can be made available to our cells, so we are increasingly likely to suffer fatigue and have to stop when we push ourselves physically. Our muscles are simply not getting enough oxygen to do their work.

Anatomical changes in our lungs compound the problem. They do not transfer as much oxygen from the outside air to the blood. Beginning at about age forty our "vital capacity," the amount of air we can move in and out of our lungs when we breathe as deeply as we can, gradually declines. By age seventy the loss in vital capacity is estimated to be about 40 percent. Once again, the result is that less oxygen reaches our muscles when they need to work at top capacity, leading to the classic symptoms of growing old—more trouble exerting ourselves, getting "winded" more easily, not being able to perform physically as we did before.

Adapting to these changes requires treading a fine line. We have to rearrange our lives to avoid situations beyond our physical limit (accept a friend's offer to drive us to the store rather than expecting to still walk the two miles), yet exert ourselves as much as we can. In fact, a major antidote to aging of the heart, and to a lesser extent the lungs, is exertion it-self—that is, exercise.

Two decades of research have demonstrated that continu-ous exercise can have a dramatic effect on cardiovascular func-tioning. For instance, when researchers compared a group of middle-aged athletes who had stopped exercising with another group who had followed a regular exercise program over thir-teen years, the first group showed the normal age-related de-cline in maximum oxygen consumption. The second group, however, actually showed increases in capacity over the years.

In other words, having once been physically active does not help much in staving off aging, but becoming and *staying* ac-tive in our middle (and later) years not only slows down nor-mal aging losses in this critical area but may even make us more fit than in our younger years.

Even though we are less able to slow normal aging in vision and hearing by changing our life-style, how we handle the small losses that occur in our senses as we age can affect the quality of our life just as dramatically.

OUR WINDOW ON THE WORLD: VISION

The eye is a marvelously complex organ, made up of a series of structures that work together to ensure that the best possible image arrives at its protected interior. The retina, the eye's in-sulated back rim, is the site of nerve endings that transform light waves into the nerve impulses carried to the brain.

As we get older, changes in several external structures cause less light to reach the retina. This dimming does not matter much in bright light, but it does matter when we need all the light we can get—in darkness. So the average person in his or her seventies tends to see well enough on a sunny day but has noticeably more difficulty seeing at night. Dim light is gloom-ier; a dark night appears pitch black.

One reason less light gets to the retina is that the lens, a clear structure toward the middle of the eye, gradually be-comes cloudier over the years. This clouding also makes see-ing in intense light more difficult; we are more likely to be blinded when a beam of light shines too directly at us. (To understand why a cloudy lens magnifies this blinding effect called glare, think what happens when you look through a slightly dirty windowpane while the sun is pouring in.)

Another change in the lens is the reason people often need bifocals by middle age. The lens is the eye's focusing apparatus. When it bends, we can see nearby objects; when it straightens out, we see objects farther away. Beginning in childhood, the lens becomes less and less flexible. This loss of flexibility means that by middle age almost everyone has more difficulty seeing close objects, and shifting one's gaze becomes more difficult. As we reach our fifties, it takes more time for objects at differing distances to come into focus.

This greater trouble in shifting gaze tends to be exacerbated by another aging change. The gray rim that develops around the pupil by our sixties causes a slight loss in peripheral vision: we cannot see quite as well as before out of the corners of our eyes.

How to Adapt

Because we need brighter light to see as well at seventy as at twenty-five, increasing the wattage of the light bulbs in your home or office may aid vision. Use incandescent lighting (regular household bulbs). Fluorescent lights (overhead tubular fixtures) may heighten seeing problems because they cause glare.

Adapting also means taking unusual care in dimly lit or glare-filled places. If you go to the movies, get there before the lights go down, or ask an usher to take you down the aisle. Go slower traversing fluorescently lit passageways. Be careful in situations where you must continually shift your gaze—such as going up or down steps. Because of poorer side vision, scan any crowded place thoroughly.

When to Get Medical Help

See a doctor immediately if you have any of these symptoms: loss or dimness of vision, eye pain, excessive discharge from the eye, double vision, or redness or swelling of the eye or eyelid. The National Institute on Aging recommends having a complete eye examination every two or three years, more often if you have diabetes or a family history of eye disease.

Some illnesses, such as glaucoma, produce symptoms only when it is too late. If they are caught in time they can be treated. Other problems, such as cataracts, can be cured by simple surgical techniques. (These common illnesses are described in table 1.) And have regular checkups to detect high blood pressure and diabetes, both of which may affect your eyes.

OUR BRIDGE TO OTHERS: HEARING

The ear also is made up of delicate outer structures and of nerve cells far within. The more external structures concentrate and amplify sound, preparing it for transmission to the brain by the delicate inner ear. By about our thirties, the nerve cells gradually begin to atrophy. The deterioration begins earlier and advances more quickly when we have been exposed to high noise levels. The cells responsible for our hearing high-pitched sounds atrophy differentially, so as we grow older we lose hearing for high tones in particular. For instance, if a tuba and a piccolo are played at an equal volume, the tuba sounds louder. Our hearing is a function of pitch, not of volume alone. Generally this loss presents problems only when it has advanced so it causes trouble in understanding conversation. But even the minor changes called "normal" require our making a few adjustments to fully enjoy being with people.

How to Adapt

The hum of background noise has a low pitch and so is more disturbing as we get older. It is more likely to drown out the closer, higher-pitched sounds we need to hear. By our seventies, hearing conversation in a noisy place is likely to be very difficult. Cocktail parties may be uncomfortable. You may wish to pass them up in favor of intimate dinners. When you go out, avoid crowded restaurants. Sit as far as possible from a noisy heater or fan. Because bare floors, low ceilings, and angled walls also magnify background noise, rooms with any of these features are bad places for a chat. (In a restaurant in my neighborhood, the combination of these three noise-magnifying features made the owners lose so much business that they were forced to completely remodel.)

Table 1   The Most Common Age-Related Eye Diseases

Cataracts
This is the normal age-related clouding of the lens described earlier carried to an extreme. The lens becomes practically opaque. Luckily, cataracts no longer need cause blindness. The defective lens is removed surgically, and either a plastic lens is implanted in the eye or special eyeglasses or contact lenses are worn.

Glaucoma
In this condition there is a buildup of fluid because a passageway that lets the fluid circulate narrows or closes up. This causes increased pressure in the eye and ultimately permanently damages the nerve cells on the retina. With early diagnosis, blindness can be prevented. Special eyedrops, medications, laser treatments, and sometimes surgery can be effective at reopening the passage. Glaucoma is called "the sneak thief of vision" because it seldom produces early symptoms, so it is important to be regularly tested for this illness in middle and later life.

Senile macular degeneration
In this disease the nerve cells in the center part of the retina (called the macula) no longer function effectively. Symptoms may include blurred vision when reading, distortion or loss of center vision, and distortion of vertical lines. Early detection is important because sometimes laser treatments can improve vision.

Diabetic retinopathy
In this complication of diabetes, the blood vessels that nourish the retina either leak fluid or grow into the eye itself and rupture, causing a serious loss of vision. Laser surgery can sometimes prevent blindness or severe loss of vision.

Retinal detachment
In this condition there is a separation between the inner and outer areas of the retina. The problem is treatable. Detached retinas can usually be surgically reattached with partial or complete restoration of vision.

My minor hearing problem used to really affect my life. At restaurants I would be reduced to silence—ashamed to ask friends to repeat themselves, afraid to risk sounding like a fool by talking when I had not really heard. It became an effort to see people. I was getting isolated and depressed. Then I hit on a simple idea: "Don't give up on people, give up on restaurants." So now even if I have to carry in cold cuts, I invite the people I want to see to my house!

If your home is noisy, you don't need to raise the ceiling or knock out walls. Consider investing in wall-to-wall carpeting. Not only does carpeting eliminate glare on bare floors and so help your vision, it also absorbs extraneous noise. To minimize the danger of another age-related problem, falling, select a low-pile rug.

Increasing the lighting in your house will also help your hearing. If you clearly see the people you are talking to, you can read lips to help make out words you do not quite hear. And because it enhances the chance of using this extra visual cue, an act as simple as always wearing your glasses may help too. Making this minor change alone can have a measurable effect.

When to Get Medical Help

People tend to put off getting help for hearing problems. The loss that is now a real impairment often has been advancing by inches over the years. No sudden symptom prompts an anxious call to the doctor. Also, having our hearing tested is not something we generally do, in contrast to a regular eye exam. Living with a problem is easy to rationalize: "It's not so bad; people are just talking too softly. Anyway, I hate the idea of a hearing aid." Hearing aids (unlike glasses) do not come in designer styles. Poor hearing (as opposed to poor vision) seems so emblematic of old age.

Foot dragging has emotional costs. Because conversation is the bridge that connects us as human beings, hearing difficulties tend to limit life even more radically than vision problems. They may affect our relationships. Personality may suffer as we strain to understand half-heard words. People may become incessant talkers to ward off having to listen, or turn taciturn and withdraw rather than risk always asking, "What did you say?" Another reaction is to become suspicious, reading plots into half-heard whispers, or to get depressed, defeated by the strain of understanding a garbled world.

If conversations are difficult to understand, or if you continually hear hissing or ringing in your ear, you need a hearing evaluation. Call your family doctor, who will either diagnose and treat your problem directly or refer you to a hearing specialist. Two types of specialists are qualified to evaluate and treat hearing difficulties: medical doctors called otolaryngologists, and audiologists—hearing specialists without an M.D. Audiologists cannot prescribe drugs or perform surgery, but they are more likely to be able to fit and sell a hearing aid.

Do not delay. If your problem is in the more external parts of the ear, it may be either curable or open to marked improvement. If you have "nerve cell damage" (the differential loss of higher-pitched sounds discussed earlier), be prepared to live with your condition. Still, a hearing aid, the sound-amplifying devices on the market (the National Association for the Deaf, in Silver Spring, Maryland, can provide a current list), or special training in understanding speech may help considerably.

Even hearing aids are no longer the badge of old age they once were. True, they have not achieved designer status, but some are now almost as good: they are invisible once in the ear.

DIGESTION

Unlike vision and hearing, many organs are involved in digestion: the esophagus, stomach, pancreas, gallbladder, liver, small intestine, and colon perform the remarkable task of breaking food into the nutrients our bodies need. Though digestive complaints are common among older people, only very minor changes normally occur in this exceedingly complex system as we grow old.

By age sixty, there is about a 25 percent reduction in the amount of saliva we produce. This loss, combined with the dental problems that occur more frequently as we age, may make it more difficult to chew foods thoroughly. It also may alter taste sensitivity slightly. Primarily because of a declining sense of smell, but also because of changes in the mouth, elderly people sometimes complain that foods either taste bland or have a disagreeable aftertaste.[7] In the stomach, less gastric juice is secreted. While this loss may affect the body's absorption of certain nutrients, it is unlikely to cause discomfort in digesting food. Changes in most of the other physiological processes involved in digestion are surprisingly hard to find. For instance, in spite of the widespread idea that constipation is almost universal in later life, waste material does not take longer to pass through the large intestine in older people.

So digestive problems are not an inevitable consequence of growing old. When they occur they either are signs of illness or are caused by changes in what we do. Poor eating habits, increased use of medications, lack of exercise, or emotional stress can interfere with digestion at any age. In later life they may wreak worse digestive havoc because they add to the small age losses that normally take place.

For instance, when we are tense we normally secrete less saliva and gastric juices. When we are anxious and older we are more likely to have problems with a dry mouth and churning stomach because the inhibiting effect of fear compounds that of age.

To ensure that your digestive system functions well, eat a balanced diet, exercise regularly, and limit emotional stress. To maintain a tip-top digestive system, National Institute on Aging experts recommend drinking alcohol sparingly and avoiding large amounts of caffeine. And if you are prone to minor stomach upsets, eat slowly and try to relax for about thirty minutes after each meal.

Constipation: The Mythic Problem
of Modest Proportions

Constipation, that so-called bane of older people, is highly overrated as a normal sign of aging. Still, the perception of a problem is strong. Older people complain to their doctors about constipation nearly five times as frequently as young adults. One reason is pure misinformation. Outdated medical thinking stressed the need for a daily bowel movement. Today's laxative ads, aimed at older consumers, beat the same ''regularity'' drum. Thus many older people are brainwashed to think ''my Metamucil'' if they do not have a bowel movement every day. But regularity just means following a regular pattern. Having a bowel movement as infrequently as twice a week can be absolutely normal if it is regular for you.

A more important sign is the quality, not the frequency, of bowel movements. Do you have difficulty passing stools? Is there pain? Are there problems such as bleeding? If these symptoms happen often, they suggest you do have a problem. Before rushing to gobble that laxative, read on.

The National Institute on Aging estimates that Americans spend $250 million a year on over-the-counter laxatives. This does more than make inroads in our pocketbooks. Heavy use of laxatives produces more constipation than it cures. Taken habitually, laxatives (and enemas) impair the body's natural emptying mechanism. We come to physically need the drug to have any bowel movement. And overuse of mineral oil, a popular laxative, may reduce the absorption of vitamins A, D, E, and K. Laxatives can also have unpleasant side effects.

If you are constipated for more than a few days, see your doctor to rule out any intestinal abnormality. Digestive-system blockages or diseases can cause constipation. Some medications are constipating, too. Then, with your physician's approval, try these remedies.

Eat high-fiber foods—fresh fruits and vegetables, whole-grain cereals and breads, and dried fruits such as prunes. Adding unprocessed bran to foods is fine but is not necessary if your diet is already high in fiber.

Drink plenty of liquids (one to two quarts a day) unless you have heart, circulatory, or kidney problems. Avoid milk. In large quantities it is constipating.

Become more physically active. Lack of physical activity is a surprisingly important cause of constipation. Begin to exercise.

Develop regular bowel habits. Regularly go to the bathroom at a certain time—for instance, after breakfast or dinner.

Never ignore the urge to defecate. Inhibiting the urge to defecate produces constipation. Although (like many people) you may feel uncomfortable having a bowel movement outside the privacy of your home, if you have a tendency to be constipated, sacrifice your delicacy for the sake of your well-being.

When to Get Medical Help

Everyone becomes constipated or has an upset stomach from time to time. However, the following symptoms are signs of real disease: (1) stomach pains that are severe, last a long time, are recurrent, or occur with shaking, chills, and cold, clammy skin; (2) vomiting blood or vomiting recurrently; (3) jaundice (yellowing of the skin) or dark, tea-colored urine; (4) pain or discomfort when swallowing food; (5) ongoing loss of appetite or unplanned weight loss; (6) diarrhea that wakes you up at night; (7) blood in your stools or coal-black stools; (8) a sudden change in your bowel habits (e.g., diarrhea or constipation) lasting more than a few days.

If you have any of these problems, call your doctor. Although our digestive system normally changes very little as the years advance, diseases of the digestive tract are not rare. In fact, they cause more hospital admissions than any other type of physical problem.

There are two errors people make in dealing with physical aging. Some stoics deny that *anything* is different and run the same ten miles on a sweltering day at age seventy as they did at twenty. Others make an equally destructive mistake: they leap to embrace the idea that aging means limitations and err on the side of doing too little.

Excess Disabilities:
The Disease of Doing Too Little

Psychologists have coined the phrase "excess disabilities" to describe what happens when people make the second type of error—when they minimize their true physical capacities and end up with disabilities they do not really have.[8] A classic case of excess disabilities occurs when Aunt Emma moves in with her daughter and within a few months can no longer cook or shop. While it seems that her health has gone into a tailspin, her physical deterioration is artificial, not real. Her loving daughter has taken over those jobs that would "strain" Mama and so has eased her entry into old age.

I have no figures on how many older people suffer from excess disabilities. But all bets are that the number is large. Though this waste of human potential can happen at age six or eighteen, conditions conspire to make older people the group most at risk. Like pregnancy, age is viewed as a delicate condition. People are told to take it easy; they are given special seats on the bus. Even someone who is running marathons at seventy is vigilant to signs of incapacity and vulnerable to excess disabilities just because of that different mind set that being older brings: "Yes, I'm fine now, but what about next week? I could have a heart attack or a stroke. I could be in a nursing home."

In a 1987 study reported in the *Journal of Gerontology*, researchers at Harvard University demonstrated that this inflated sense of physical vulnerability does tend to hit us in later life.[9] They asked 480 people aged forty-five to eighty-nine this question: "In general, how would you rate your physical health? Would you say it is excellent, good, fair, or poor?" Then they compared the answers to a variety of objective indexes—hospital stays, diagnoses, health as rated by physicians. When they divided their subjects into two groups, middle-aged people (forty-five to sixty-four) and older people (sixty-five and over), the researchers discovered that age itself produced physical pessimism. People with identical objective health ratings were more likely to label themselves in worse health if they were over sixty-five.

The lesson of this study is that when we are older we must take special care not to succumb to this self-fulfilling prophecy: "Age means incapacity." To guard against excess disabilities, never accept health advice based on your age alone: "At eighty no person should still be playing tennis"; "You're seventy, so isn't it time to give up jogging that daily mile?" Remember, everyone's body ages differently. If you are convinced you are capable of doing something and your physician agrees, have confidence. Provided you are sensitive to your body's signals, you are the best judge of what you can do.

Make the saying "one swallow doesn't make a summer" your motto. Tell yourself "my age" is the last, not the first, explanation to accept when something goes physically or mentally wrong. Saying a symptom is due to "old age" is the same thing as saying nothing can be done. Consider any physical change for the worse curable until proved otherwise.

Here are some times to be on special guard against excess disabilities, and ways to implement this new "it's not me" mind set.

You are kept from doing what you physically can do. When any barrier impedes independent functioning, people are especially vulnerable to developing excess disabilities. The barrier might be another person—a well-meaning "helper" who takes over jobs you can do for yourself. Or the impediment might be truly physical: your living conditions themselves may magnify any minor limitations you have.

For example, because climbing the hill to his apartment building is difficult, Mr. Jones does not go out as much. Yesterday, when he did leave the house, it was much harder to walk around the block. If he lived in the building at the bottom of the hill, he would be walking to the store every day. Standing on her feet for a long time is a strain, so Mrs. Walker lets her husband take over the cooking. Soon she is even more physically depleted, unable to stand at all. In both cases, minor difficulties are being transformed into life-crippling problems because the environment is fostering incapacity instead of promoting an independent life.

The solution. If you feel this problem fits you, try this approach: (1) Home in on exactly what is keeping you from functioning up to your potential (standing too long by the stove; reaching for food and seasonings). (2) Think of several possible solutions to each problem. (To avoid standing too long, I could bring a chair into the kitchen; cook meals not requiring elaborate preparation. To avoid reaching, I could rearrange the shelves more conveniently; ask my husband to set out the dinner ingredients *but not take over everything.*) (3) Decide which courses of action are most feasible and implement them. If you have problems in carrying out a plan, try a backup. Don't give up until your environment brings out your physical best.

You have recently been ill or have had a frightening symptom. It is easy to develop excess disabilities after a temporary medical scare. Even though the problem is a passing one, the person thinks, "I am old." So it seems only logical to assume the body has permanently broken down.

For instance, one hot day a man gets dizzy on the tennis court. He concludes, "This is it. I'm just too old to play anymore." But the correct lesson should be "Play, but avoid sweltering days." Or a woman falls walking down the steps of her building after she has been in bed for a week with a fever and decides she will never go out alone again. Or since his heart attack Mr. Smith has given up sex completely, even though the doctor gives him a clean bill of health.

The solution. If this difficulty applies to you, visit your doctor for a checkup and reassurance. Then start regaining your confidence slowly. Play a short volley of tennis on a cool day and gradually build up. Take a friend and be very careful the next time you negotiate those steps. Going slowly at first will help ensure that you don't have any new symptoms, and it will let you begin believing in your body again.

You regularly take medications. Side effects of medication often mimic classic symptoms of "old age." Sometimes adverse reactions appear days or weeks after you begin taking a drug, making it difficult to connect the physical change with the medicine. Disabling side effects are more likely to be endured rather than questioned in later life, because they are misinterpreted as the new "old" me.

For months an unmentionable problem made me reluctant to venture out. While shopping or visiting a friend, I would feel a gooey sensation between my legs. Imagine my dismay when I confessed to my daughter and this was her response: "That's terrible, Mom, but what do you expect at eighty-five?" I could not accept the idea that I was doomed to diapers, and so I tried frantically to link my problem to another cause. I came up with the idea that my trouble had started after I began taking my heart pill. I called my doctor, we tried another medicine, and my "old age" incontinence was gone.

How common are drug-caused excess disabilities? We can get an inkling from the iceberg's tip. From 12 to 17 percent of all hospital admissions for the elderly are caused by adverse drug effects.[10] If the rate of severe reactions is this high, the incidence of moderate side effects must be many times higher. Sometimes we willingly accept an unpleasant symptom as the price a drug exacts for saving our lives. But sometimes we suffer needlessly out of ignorance, when another medicine would work just as well or when *no* drug might leave us better off.

Using Medications Safely

Although they are lifesavers, medications are a double-edged sword in later life. Because of age-related physiological losses, most are less efficiently metabolized and excreted. A dose tolerated well at age twenty is more likely to be toxic at sixty-five. At the same time, at sixty-five or eighty people are more likely to be taking several medicines. Because people differ so much physically, drug companies can devise only general guidelines for how high a dose is "too much" at a given age. To minimize the chance of adverse drug reactions, the National Institute on Aging advises taking these steps when a new medication is prescribed.[11]

Tell your doctor exactly which other over-the-counter and prescription drugs you are using. Also tell your physician if you have previously had any adverse reactions to certain medications.

Ask about the medication's side effects. Don't be afraid you will develop the symptoms just by hearing about them. Being ill informed is not bliss.

Be vigilant to unusual symptoms during the first few weeks after beginning the drug. If symptoms appear, report them promptly.

Regularly reevaluate the need for the medication. Because new information about drugs and older people is continually coming to light, periodically review your medication regimen with your doctor.

One reason for the high rate of toxic side effects is memory lapses. A woman forgets she already took her morning pill and takes a double dose. A man samples that delicious new cheese at a party, forgetting it is on his list of "drug contraindications." Errors related to taking or not taking medicines multiply when people are taking more than one drug. For instance, in a recent survey of patients at a geriatric clinic, the average person failed to remember 46 percent of the medications listed in his or her chart.[12]

If your drug regimen is at all complicated, remembering what to take when, what foods to avoid, and what medicine has or has not been taken that day can strain the capacities of an Einstein. You must rely on memory aids to help you out. Here are two useful ones.[13]

Post a list of the drugs you are taking next to the cabinet where you keep your medicines. Your record should show the name of each drug, the doctor who prescribed it, and the times of day for taking it. Next to each drug, include a week's spaces. For instance, a listing might look like this: Drug X, Dr. Prudent, 3 × a day: Monday ____, Tuesday ____, etc. Attach a pencil and check off the doses in the appropriate spaces as you take them. Keep a copy of your list in your wallet so you can do the same when you are out. Before you go to bed Sunday evening, erase the previous week's record and begin again.

Or buy a pillbox with seven compartments and fill it with the week's pills each Sunday evening before you go to bed. If you take a yellow pill three times a day and a red pill twice, place all five daily pills in each of the seven compartments. Then if you are unsure whether you took a certain pill, you will know just by counting how many of that day's supply are left.

Either of these methods will tell you if you have already taken a particular pill. To remember to take your medicine in the first place, anchor your pill taking to another habitual activity. For instance, if one pill must be taken three times a day and the other twice, take them with meals—one at breakfast, lunch, and dinner and the other at breakfast and dinner. Eventually, swallowing your pill will become so much a part of mealtime that you will automatically think "my medicine" as you take your first bite.

As a fail-safe measure, put your medication record where you have to see it. If you take pills with meals, tape your list to the refrigerator or leave your pillbox in the middle of the kitchen counter. If you take pills at bedtime and on awakening, place your record in an eye-catching place next to the bed. Also put drug-interaction warnings in an eye-catching place. If you must avoid a long list of substances while on a given pill, post the list in your kitchen and in your medicine cabinet. Keep a copy in your wallet to refer to when you go out.

These techniques are not too bothersome. Once in place they require just the ounce of forethought it takes to look both ways before crossing the street. Both habits may be equally lifesaving.

Sticking to Good Health Habits

In addition to guarding against excess disabilities, the research shows that prevention is crucial. Exercising, not smoking, and adhering to good health habits are doubly important as the years advance. But the key is consistency, continuing a life-extension program for life. And the rewards of lighting an after-dinner cigarette or living on cake are more immediate and so have a powerful pull. But psychologists think the idea that people abandon their attempts to live healthfully because they lack willpower is wrong. Quitters are simply people who use poor strategies. The way they put their resolutions into practice makes it difficult *not* to backslide. Taking these steps will help you stick to a health improvement plan.

Make sure your plan is medically sound. For instance, more precautions are needed to exercise safely when you are over sixty-five. You must build up more slowly and take special care not to push yourself too hard. If you want to lose weight, the same cautions apply. Choose a diet that is gradual, healthful, and reasonable. Crash dieting or unorthodox diets are more likely to shorten life than extend it. Consult an expert to devise a plan that fits your needs and capacities (e.g., visit a registered dietitian), or ask your family doctor for guidance. If you have gotten your plan from a book, get your doctor's blessing before going ahead.

Determine what will make sticking to your plan easiest. Devise a few possible strategies and write your ideas down. Ask yourself: "What is impeding my following through now?" Are you eating cake all day because you live alone and it's too much trouble to fix a good meal? Is there nothing but bread in the house because it's hard to get to the store? If so, would it help to buy more food less often so you can prepare a week's meals on one day and freeze them? Would you exercise more comfortably alone, to a tape or a favorite record, or along with a television program? Or would it help if you paid money and felt forced to attend a class regularly? If sit-ups and stretches are too boring to contemplate, is there a sport you might really enjoy?

Carry out each choice mentally to arrive at the best alternative. For instance, you might think, "I would feel best if I went to a class, but I would have to go to one nearby. I might have a problem if the class were filled with eighteen-year-olds. I think I'll see if the local senior center has a group."

Write down a place, number of hours, and time(s) for carrying out your plan. Make a specific, rigid schedule for following through: "I must sit at the table and eat three times a day. From 5:00 to 6:00 I'll prepare dinner and the next day's lunch." "At 4:00 P.M. I'll do twenty minutes of exercise to a tape." "On Monday, Wednesday, and Friday I'll take that beginner's swim class at the Y."

Making a schedule instead of having a vague intention forces us to confront the sensation of success or failure at a certain time. Since we are creatures of habit, when we do anything regularly at the same time and place it eventually becomes automatic. The pattern takes on a life of its own, and soon we feel vaguely out of sorts, or downright deprived, if something happens and we cannot do what we always do.

Reward yourself regularly for sticking to the plan. Until your resolution becomes the mental equivalent of brushing your teeth and you are motivated to keep going just by how much better you feel, build in external rewards for not falling off the wagon. Here too, make a schedule. Do something definite every week or two to congratulate yourself: go to the theater, buy a dress, or simply enjoy an afternoon spent at home with a good book or visiting an old friend you rarely see. Rewarding yourself at close intervals is better than planning something big six months or a year away. It is too hard at the outset to contemplate following through for a lifetime, but almost anyone can stick to a plan for a week at a time.

In taking more control over your physical fate, be encouraged by this fact: there is no one-to-one relation between the results of medical tests—of vision or hearing or any other physical ability—and how a person functions. Some people with minor problems are disabled; others with more severe losses do fine. Since how we function, not our score on a test of lung function, is what is important, the message is clear. Apart from extending your life, what you do today to improve your health will have an immediate payoff on the most important index of how old you are—how old you act.

For More Information

POPULAR GUIDES TO GOOD HEALTH

American Association for Retired Persons. *Strategies for Good Health*. Washington, D.C.: AARP, Health Advocacy Services Program Department, 1985.
Booklet giving general information about health-promoting strategies such as exercise and diet. Also offers advice on choosing a doctor, getting a second opinion, and using medical services wisely. Write to the AARP at 1909 K Street N.W., Washington, D.C. 20049.

De Vries, H., and D. Hales. *Fitness after Fifty*. New York: Scribner's, 1982. Book describing how to exercise appropriately when older.

National Institute on Aging and Pfizer Pharmaceuticals. *Help Yourself to Good Health*. Rockville, Md.: National Institute on Aging, 1985.

The Age Pages are fact sheets on normal aging and health care published by the National Institute on Aging. *Help Yourself to Good Health* is a compilation of the Age Pages. These topics and others are addressed: normal age-related changes in vision, hearing, and other systems; information about the safe use of medicines, optimal diet, the value of exercise, and finding good medical care. Write to the National Institute on Aging Public Affairs Office, Room 6C10, Federal Building, 7550 Wisconsin Avenue, Bethesda, Maryland 20892 for free copies.

ACADEMICALLY ORIENTED PUBLICATIONS

Department of Health, Education, and Welfare (United States Public Health Service). National Institute on Aging Science Writing Seminar Series.

Collection of articles on biological theories of aging, the Baltimore
study and other important findings in the biology of aging. Write
to the NIA Public Affairs Office for copies (see address above).

Shock, N., and associates. *Normal Human Aging: The Baltimore
Longitudinal Study of Aging.* Rockville, Md.: National Institute
on Aging, 1984.

Describes the findings of the Baltimore study as of 1984. Difficult
but interesting. Write to the NIA Public Affairs Office for free copies (see address above).

2

THE MIND

Going back to college and being an A student does little to ease my feelings about my learning ability at this stage of life. I can't help feeling that I'm at a basic disadvantage because of my age. True, I'm a bit better now. At first, when I read an assignment and didn't absorb it the first time—pure panic. Now I'm able to reassure myself a bit, but I still feel I have to work twice as hard to measure up. I'll be frank, this is the worst fear associated with aging—always being conscious of your mental state. Now when I forget something or miss an appointment, I cannot forget it. The thoughts keep coming: Is this the beginning of senility? Can I really still trust myself? I know I'm not unusual. Most of us feel that by magic birthday sixty-five we must be mentally worse off. At the back of our minds is the terror of Alzheimer's disease.

This woman is a wonderful student, but success does not touch her fear. She shrugs off A+ work as due to extra effort and misinterprets normal forgetting as mental decline. Her oversensitivity is understandable. From childhood we have been taught to judge old people by a harsher mental standard, seeing evidence of basic confusion in even benign mistakes.

Psychologists Judith Rodin of Yale University and Ellen Langer of Harvard University demonstrated this bias by filming three actors aged twenty, fifty, and seventy reading the same speech.[1] Scattered through the ten-minute monologue were a few comments such as "Yesterday I forgot my keys." People of different ages then watched the film of either the young, middle-aged, or older actor and were asked to write an essay telling what he was like. Those who saw the seventy-year-old frequently described him as forgetful. None of those who had seen the identical words read by the middle-aged person or young adult mentioned poor memory.

Unfortunately, the older people who saw the film were just as likely as the younger viewers to see the seventy-year-old as slipping mentally, and they were even more likely to evaluate him in a negative way.

This is just one of many studies demonstrating that we are primed to look for signs of mental confusion in older people.[2] When someone is seventy (or sixty-five, or eighty) we do interpret normal forgetting in an exaggerated, more ominous light. But Rodin and Langer's finding that the victims of this prejudice practice it too is particularly distressing. If older people leap just as readily to misjudge someone their own age, don't they turn the same overharsh judgments inward? How many people are haunted for days by the idea "I'm getting senile" just because they are over sixty-five and have misplaced their keys?

Beware of self-diagnosing your memory. If you think it has seriously declined, you are probably not right. Psychologist Robin West of the University of Florida and her colleagues gave women ranging in age from sixty-five to ninety a variety of memory tests and also tested their emotional state—their anxiety and depression, their satisfaction with life.[3] The researchers then asked the women how bad or good they felt their memory was: Do you have problems remembering names? Do you remember better than your friends? Do you feel your memory is good or poor?

The women who believed they had a poor memory did just as well as anyone else on the actual memory tests. But they were more fearful and less happy. In this 1984 study, West demonstrated what other psychologists have found: older people are not accurate judges of their memory. They tend to feel their memory is bad not so much when it is bad as when they are *feeling* bad.[4]

But even if we may not be good at self-diagnosis, isn't it true that as we get older not just our memory but our overall mental sharpness declines? We do gradually lose brain cells. Shouldn't that have an effect on our ability to think? Before looking at the research on memory and aging, let's consider that more basic question. Do we get less intelligent as the years advance?

Aging and IQ:
Why the Experts Steered Us Wrong

Imagine you are a first-time tennis player and are competing against someone in regular training. Your opponent not only has been practicing almost daily for years, but also is a self-confident master of the rules. As your nightmare ends, you lose and then are blamed not for putting yourself in such a ridiculous situation but for being much worse than he is in your basic aptitude for the game.

This is exactly what used to happen to older people when they took intelligence tests. Totally unused to being tested (having been out of school for years) and anxious about their minds anyway, they were then compared with younger, more skilled test takers. When the older people did not measure up, their poorer showing was labeled intellectual decline owing to advancing age.

For close to a quarter of a century, since the standard test of adult intelligence (the Wechsler Adult Intelligence Scale) was developed in the early 1940s, this error was made repeatedly. Psychologists believed that our mental capacities begin a general downslide starting as early as our twenties. Few people recognized that the basic logic was faulty, that older generations might test poorly in part because they were out of practice—not knowing how to take tests efficiently, being out of school too long, and having far fewer years of schooling than their children (or grandchildren). Everyone was compared as if they were equal. Few people noticed that the test-taking dice were heavily loaded in favor of the young.

Then in the early 1970s psychologist K. Walter Schaie and his colleagues published the results of a fourteen-year study. These University of Washington researchers tested hundreds of adults three times, in 1956, 1963, and 1970. They had developed a way of roughly determining the contribution of ''experience and education'' to the so-called age loss in IQ. Using their formula, they conclusively demonstrated that much of the decline in IQ scores was indeed due to these extraneous factors.[5] The idea that our intelligence goes steadily downhill after our twenties is just not true.

Actually, our logic is wrong when we label people intelligent based just on their scores on the standard intelligence test. Most experts now feel there are separate types of intelligence. (For instance, psychologist Howard Gardner of Harvard University feels there may be as many as twenty independent "intelligences.") IQ tests measure only a limited set—the intellectual skills needed for doing well in school. They test our ability to come up with the right answer, not our ability to understand or get along with people, our creativity or wisdom, our street smarts, or our artistic gifts. Because of this, a person who tests at the genius level on an IQ test is likely to be an A + student. But his friend who scores average may be the genius at life.

This misinterpretation of the meaning of intelligence tests mainly hurts children. They are most likely to be ranked and categorized as "smart," "average," or "slow" by an IQ score. But it also affects our understanding of older people who have to be tested. Because the test does not do a good job of measuring the qualities that make up intelligence in the real world, an adult's score is particularly likely to inadequately reflect true mental capacities. Realizing this, psychologists are beginning to develop better tests of life intelligence, measures that will capture the wisdom, good sense, and balanced perspective on living that are the true signs of intelligence in the classroom of life.

What skills make up real-world intelligence? At the 1986 meeting of the American Psychological Association, Gisela Labouvie of Wayne State University and Fredda Blanchard-Fields of Louisiana State University provided some clues.[6] Both psychologists believe that real-world intelligence does not involve picking out *the* correct answer to an abstract problem, which is what the standard IQ test asks us to do, but thinking in a different way. In school people who can solve academic problems are considered the intelligent ones. But real-world problems often have no clear-cut right or wrong solutions. Making intelligent life decisions means being sensitive to the many perspectives involved in issues and integrating them to arrive at answers that are "wise" rather than absolutely correct. It also means going beyond rational logic in making decisions. People who have real-world intelligence are socially smart. They have a gift for understanding other human beings; they can intuit the emotional (sometimes irrational) logic of the heart. Test your life intelligence by answering this problem:

John is known to be a heavy drinker, especially when he goes to parties. Mary, John's wife, warns him that if he gets drunk one more time she will leave him. Tonight John is out at an office party and comes home drunk. Does Mary leave John?

When Labouvie asks young adolescents this question, their answer is a rigid yes. "Mary said she would leave, so of course she does." People in their thirties and forties are sensitive that the issue is not black-and-white. They think about the pros and cons—for Mary, for John, for their children. They know that a simple yes or "she should" may not be the best response. Their answers are more intelligent because they are more attuned to the realities of life.

A real-world intelligence test will probably measure how we think about common dilemmas like this one. Until psychologists develop this test, though, we must be content to measure intelligence mainly by the single-answer IQ test we have always used, oriented to academic logic. It too can tell us some very important things.

The Wechsler Adult Intelligence Scale is divided into two parts. The first part tests our fund of knowledge—vocabulary, ability to calculate, factual information we have absorbed. The second part of the test measures on-the-spot analytical skills—putting together puzzles or blocks to make the right design, arranging pictures so they "tell a story" or transcribing unfamiliar symbols. A premium is placed on speed; the tasks in this half of the test are timed.

As people get older they do very differently on the two parts. They do relatively well on the first half of the test. Beginning quite early (in the twenties), they do more and more poorly on the second part as the years pass, for each section of the test measures a basically different intellectual skill.

Psychologists call the type of intelligence mainly measured by the first half of the test crystallized intelligence. It is the amount of knowledge we have stored in our brain. In contrast, a very different skill is measured by the second half—our ability to come up with the correct solution to a totally unfamiliar abstract problem in the shortest possible time. This basic intellectual skill is called fluid intelligence.

As we get older, provided we remain active and involved in life, our crystallized intelligence tends to increase, because the rate of new learning normally exceeds the rate at which we forget. There are two situations when forgetting tends to surpass the volume of new information we absorb—illness and withdrawal from life. If we are very sick or pull back emotionally from the world, we are not motivated to learn new things, so what goes out exceeds what comes in, and crystallized intelligence declines.[7]

This finding about aging and IQ has been demonstrated repeatedly: people who have a complex life-style, who have compelling interests, activities, and—just as important— meaningful, stimulating contact with other people tend, if anything, to increase their scores on the first part of the IQ test.[8] When crystallized intelligence does decline after age fifty, or seventy, it is often because our lives have become less stimulating—through illness, or lack of opportunity, or losing interest in learning new things.

Unfortunately, the findings are not so upbeat for fluid intelligence. This type of intelligence does begin to decline rapidly and quite early, by our late twenties or early thirties. The main reason is loss of speed. As we get older we get slower, not so much in how fast we move, but in how fast we think. The gradual loss in fluid intelligence begins right after we reach adulthood. But it only becomes a real problem in some limited situations by about midlife.

For instance, an air-traffic controller may notice his performance at work getting worse by his early forties. His job depends on split-second decisions, and so his skill is likely to be affected a good deal by age. Luckily, relatively little of what most of us do depends on analyzing ever-changing information very fast. The few minutes or seconds of decision-making time we lose is usually more than offset by our crystallized intelligence—the knowledge and experience we also accumulate over the years.

Let's illustrate the fluid/crystallized difference by placing odds on a twenty-five-year-old lawyer versus his sixty-year-old opposing attorney to win a court case. The young lawyer, with his fluid intelligence at its peak, could reason and write faster. But our betting odds should be on the seasoned veteran. He is at a clear advantage because of his greater crystallized intelligence, his years of experience in what to research and how best to argue the case.

A study of 150 members of the 1973–74 Vermont legislature makes just this point. Although the younger legislators proposed about twice as many bills, an older legislator's chance of getting a given proposal passed was more than twice as great. The slower production rate of the older legislators was easily counterbalanced by the gift that being older conferred: knowing how to prepare legislation better and understanding which types of bills would pass.[9]

There is a physical basis for our gradual loss of fluid intelligence. Our brain cells (neurons) do not send signals and communicate with one another as quickly as they once did. So it takes us more time to process information, from a few milliseconds to a few seconds longer depending on our age, our individual capacities, and the complexity of what we are asked to do. But though this decline is biological, there is an encouraging physical basis for the fact that crystallized intelligence can increase almost to the end of life.

The Brain Grows in
Middle and Later Life

In a study published in *Science*, Steven Buell and Paul Coleman of Rochester University compared the neurons of a group of people dying at about eighty with those of people dying at age fifty and a group who had died while suffering from dementia (the average age of this last group was about seventy-five).[10] They were astonished to find that the neurons of the normal elderly had many more interconnections than those of the middle-aged people they examined. This finding of more neural branches in the older brains is crucial because it is the number of *connections* between cells, not the number of cells, that is a main physical basis of learning and memory. Yes, it is true that we gradually lose brain cells as we get older. But the remaining cells compensate for this loss by growing more branches. And at least by the index of number of branches, we may actually develop "superior" brains.

In fact, in this study the dendrites—the branching part of the neuron—of the people with Alzheimer's disease were the most different from those of the normal people. Their dendrites were the shortest, emphasizing that instead of being normal aging, senility is abnormal indeed. (As I will describe in chapter 9, the brain cells of people who have Alzheimer's disease look like dying trees; first their dendrites shrivel, and then the whole cell wastes away to a stump.)

At the same 1986 meeting of the American Psychological Association where a real-world intelligence test was being discussed, Coleman presented his latest research on our remarkable ability to grow more brain. He measured dendrite growth in a section of the brain called the dentate gyrus in four groups: young adults, middle-aged people, old people (aged seventy), and very old people (aged ninety). From these calculations he estimates that on average we may "grow" 3 million millimeters more dendrites per year in middle and later life, an increase more than enough to compensate for the cells we lose. The growth in dendrites occurred in Coleman's middle-aged subjects and the seventy-year-olds, but in his very old subjects (the ninety-year-olds) it did stop. So we do eventually lose this wonderful mechanism for compensating for lost brain cells, but only if we live to a very old age.[11]

Coleman hypothesizes that the biochemical message to grow new dendrites switches on automatically as brain cells are lost. But a fascinating set of studies done by neuropsychologist Marian Diamond of the University of California suggests that how much growth occurs is also affected by what we do.[12]

In her first studies, Diamond raised rats in what she called an enriched environment. They grew up in cages full of various objects, were regularly played with, and were given new things to explore. As adults the animals reared in this way had heavier brains and also acted more intelligent. The cortex (the top part of the brain) was thicker, and they ran a maze much better than rats raised under normal laboratory conditions.

This research has implications for the way we raise children. A mentally stimulating early environment may increase our brain growth in the first years of life and so set us up to be intelligent adults. But what about the years after childhood? Does the environment have any effect on the aging brain?

Diamond's latest studies suggest it does. Older rats put in the same enriched environment also developed a thicker cortex and showed more signs of intelligence. The effect was surprisingly similar to that found in the young animals.

When we combine this animal research with the finding that crystallized intelligence increases when people lead a complex life, everything indicates that stimulating contact with the world is crucial to keeping our intelligence fine-tuned. During our working years, the need for an adequately stimulating life is likely to take care of itself. Having a job and raising a family are challenges that (often) force us to use our brains. But as we reach retirement age, we may less often be forced to exercise our mental muscles. We must more actively search out an enriched outer life. If we allow our interest in the world and living to erode greatly, we can expect to pay a price. Not only may we seem less intelligent, but our brain itself could change.

Developing a Stimulating Life

If you feel your life needs enrichment, here are some steps to take.

Make a list of the things you are most interested in or most like to do. Your interests do not have to be intellectual, but they should be heartfelt. Almost any activity except "sleeping" or "thinking about nothing" could legitimately be on your list. If you cannot think of an activity in your life now that might really excite you, try to remember what used to interest you and list those things.

Carefully examine how you might do the things on your list in a way that enhances active involvement in the world. If you like to read, would you be interested in going back to school? If you like children, could you volunteer at a local day-care center or call your neighbors and tell them you are available to baby-sit? If your most satisfying interest was your career and you are retired, would you want to find part-time work in your former field, or could you find volunteer work related to your former job?

If you feel anxious about jumping headlong into new waters or are afraid you won't be able to carry your plan through, use this technique: Make a timetable for doing that new thing step by little step. Do something toward your goal every day. Reward yourself for any emotionally hard advance. Know that your thinking can become better just from the exhilaration of making a plan. Something as simple as having the courage to make that first call can have a surprisingly widespread effect. All of a sudden we become transformed from cowards to people who just might be more in control than we thought. Each successive act is likely to get easier. There is indeed an emotional ripple effect. Soon what took bravery and effort is—provided you have chosen correctly—transformed into pure fun.

But are activities all we need to exercise our minds? The answer is probably no.

I do less with people, so my memory does less. I can't often afford the theater, ballet, or movies, so TV must substitute. The problem is not that TV is less intellectual, but that you are more likely to watch it alone. Without activities that require a companion, the stimulating exchange of viewpoints is lost. Most hobbies are for do-it-yourselfers, so again a person is engaged in solitary work—no discussion, no competition, no joy at exposing, by talking to someone else, what the mind can really do—only my own determination. No help for memory there. No, I'm not less intelligent than I used to be. I just have less chance to be intelligent because I am more often alone.

This woman is too negative about what life can offer. But her insight that having a sharp mind depends on being with other people may be scientifically sound. This is the conclusion we can draw from a study published in the mid-1970s in the *British Journal of Psychiatry*. Peter Brook and his colleagues compared the thinking of nursing-home residents exposed to memory-stimulating props such as newspapers, interesting objects, and constant reminders of the day and place with the memory of others who were stimulated socially—an interested person just spent time talking to them. Only the memory of those who were talked to improved.[13] Human communication was the brain-cell medicine that worked!

So in preference to solitary activities it is better to choose something involving others. But this advice applies only if being lonely is a special problem for you. In a 1985 study, Reed Larson of the University of Chicago and his co-workers charted the number of hours per day people of various ages spent alone.[14] They found that in later life we tend to spend more time by ourselves than we did in our earlier years. (For instance, the older people in this study who were married spent about 40 percent of their waking hours alone). Being alone does not bother us. But this is true only if we have the choice to be with others. Larson's older subjects who had no spouse or other close relationship chafed at the hours they spent in solitude. Loneliness happens when there is no one we care about whom we can immediately call. It is a feeling that is just as painful, sharp, and important to change at any age.

You should not accept loneliness as the inevitable price of being older, even if you are living alone. Despite the idea that loneliness is rampant among the elderly, in a nationwide Harris poll taken in 1981 people over sixty-five did not report being lonely more often than younger adults.[15]

If you are lonely and have compelling interests, use them to enrich yourself and increase your circle of friends. Instead of painting at home, try enrolling in an art class. Rather than exercising alone, look into joining a group. Conversation will not be such a problem, because you can discuss your shared passion with the people you meet. And because you do have this common interest there is a chance you'll find a true kindred soul.

At the same time, monitor the events in your week to see how much contact with other people you do have. If you decide you are alone too much, plan to increase your social activities by a definite (but achievable) number of hours each week. Ruthlessly apply the same list-making strategy you used for interests to selecting friends. Rank people from "those I like most" to "those I least prefer." Try each day to make a call or two to arrange a date. Concentrate on people near the top of your list. You don't need to invite someone to go to the theater or an expensive restaurant. People will be flattered if you ask them for tea or a stroll in the park. But you must *want* to be with the person you choose. Meaningless social engagements (or activities) will leave you feeling it is more satisfying to do nothing. The essence of staying intelligent is to arrange an outer life that fulfills your inner preferences and desires.

What About That Other Influence on the Mind—the Body?

As I mentioned earlier, there is a connection between our physical state and our mental sharpness. When people are sick, their IQ scores tend to decline.[16] Illness saps us of the energy to think clearly. Some diseases—a heart condition or arteriosclerosis or hypertension, for instance—may even impair the blood supply and nutrients that get to our brain.[17]

If you are one of the many people with a chronic condition, do not read this information as your intellectual epitaph. Provided you do not have a brain illness such as Alzheimer's disease (see chap. 9), the direct effect your disease may have on your clarity of mind is likely to be minor. Its indirect impact may be marked—being sick keeps you from having a stimulating life. When we are focusing on our aches and pains or are confined by illness to looking at four walls, it is difficult to be intelligent. It is the way disease constricts our life that makes us less mentally quick.

If you are sick, take special care to remain as mentally active as possible. Reread the discussion of excess disabilities in chapter 1. Ask yourself: "Is my illness restricting my life to an excessive degree?" "How can I be more active in the world and so improve my thinking in spite of my condition?" Read the section in chapter 10 on living with disability. Search out any device that will help you be more physically independent.

By what hook or crook can you get to that art class or lecture? If you cannot get there, is there a way of doing the same intellectually enriching activity at home? Evaluate your medications with your doctor; many drugs have a dulling effect. Have you become more dizzy or drowsy since beginning that pill? If so, could you change to another or reduce the dose?

Our physical state can be a damper to staying mentally active, but it is not an insurmountable one. Many of the world's masterpieces have been fired in the crucible of physical suffering: The example of Beethoven and Michelangelo producing their finest work in their years of declining health shows that even in an unsound body, the mind can soar.

Remembering, Forgetting, and Getting Older

Studies show that most people over sixty-five feel their memory has gotten worse, and scientific research corroborates their belief. Older people as a group do get worse scores than the young on memory tests. But knowing this fact is not enough. The question is why. To understand the issues, it is important to get a picture of what memory involves.

The way we have a memory can be conceptualized as occurring in separate steps. Information seems to pass through a three-step sequence (or three storage bins) in the process of becoming "a memory."[18] The first step or storage area is a momentary snapshot of everything we see or hear that remains in the brain for roughly one second. We know this brief mental photograph of everything is there and then goes away because of a classic experiment.[19] This group of lines is flashed on a screen and then quickly disappears:

	Previous instructions to subject
A C 2 P D	High tone means read this line
L 3 U Z K	Medium tone means read this line
S 2 7 1 A	Low tone means read this line

The person watching the screen has been told that a buzzer sounding in the prearranged way described above means to repeat as much as possible of the appropriate line. If the signal goes off within one second after the lines have disappeared, performance is often flawless. Almost every item is likely to be correct. But a signal only milliseconds later than that may mean abject failure; the person will recall one or two letters or numbers at most. The reason is that in that instant our snapshot has faded; the first memory step has already dissipated.

This is all to the good, since we need to remember only a fraction of the welter of information that continually impinges on our senses. So it is just the tiny fragment of this first photographic image that we really attend to that gets to the next step or bin, short-term memory. Short-term memory is the amount of information we can hold in our minds at a given time. This turns out to be about seven separate words or numbers or items.

We see the limit of short-term memory vividly when we get a telephone number from information and immediately make the call. We know by experience that we can dial the seven-digit number without having to write it down and that memory will not fail us provided the phone rings. If we get a busy signal, though, and have to try again, memory mysteriously fades. We have reached the twenty-second limit of this second memory phase.

To really remember the phone number or anything else, we must transfer what is in short-term memory to the most important system, long-term memory. Long-term memory is what we really mean when we think of memory, the sum total of things that we can recall from our past. Although emotionally charged events such as our wedding days or the births of our children are effortlessly embedded in this possibly permanent huge memory warehouse, often getting something into and out of long-term memory takes effort. We have to learn (or get in) what we want to remember in the first place. We have to retrieve (or get out) what we have learned at the right time. So while the word remembering means "getting something out," the important first step in having a memory of something is getting it in. If we haven't put the items we want into our warehouse in the first place, we will never be able to find and retrieve them. Learning something adequately is crucial to remembering.

The happy news is that getting older has virtually no effect on the first two memory steps. But older people on average do worse than the young on tests of the most important system, long-term memory. We now know that the difficulty could be either poor learning or poor recall (not being able to get out things already in our warehouse). Where does the basic problem lie?

Many people would probably guess poor recall, saying, "My brain is so crowded with memories already that I have trouble getting that phone number or name out at the appropriate time. I know I know it, and it is still there somewhere, I just can't find it now." Or they might put their difficulty in a more negative way: "Isn't it true that because we lose brain cells, some memories once put into storage have been totally lost?"

The explanation of an overcrowded brain is not quite accurate, but we are noticing something that may really occur. As we grow older it may take longer to get a memory out, not because our storehouse is jammed to the rafters, but because of the age-related decline in thinking speed. Slower thinking probably accounts for at least part of the panicky feeling that our memory is less sharp. We confuse the fact that it takes a bit longer to remember something with the idea that there is something basically wrong with the whole system.

Unless a person is truly suffering from an illness such as Alzheimer's disease, I am happy to say that brain-cell loss is unlikely to be the reason for not remembering something. You probably can't retrieve the memory you want not because it has been totally lost, but because it never fully got in in the first place. Many memory researchers studying aging now believe that the main reason some of us do not remember things as well when we get older is that we simply haven't adequately memorized (or learned) what we want to remember. The problem is not so much getting things out of storage as putting them in.

It isn't so much that our basic ability to learn gets worse past age sixty or seventy; it's often that for a variety of reasons we get out of practice. If we are retired, our bread and butter no longer depends on our mastering that new information or remembering to make those critical calls. So the pressure to keep learning and remembering is off; the training that sharpens memory is no longer there. Suddenly we are aware of forgetting more. A main reason is that we have lost our memorization skills. Having a good memory depends on being able to concentrate and also requires effective memorization techniques.

We all have noticed that some events seem indelibly fixed in our brains while most of life's experiences quickly fade. The main characteristic of the things we always remember is their meaningful quality. Events that are emotionally important are learned the best. The first prerequisite for learning anything well, then, is to make it vivid and emotionally meaningful. When your job depended on remembering a customer's name, there was no problem with making it emotionally important. Now it may help to use special strategies to charge yourself up.

Mnemonic techniques are ways of making things that are hard to remember (such as names) emotionally vivid. Researchers have shown that older people rarely use these special techniques, but usually just rely on rote "memorization" in the memory laboratory.[20] This makes it doubly hard to embed things securely in the brain. If older people are asked to remember something that is already personally meaningful, or if they are taught to use mnemonic strategies to *make* meaning out of what they are learning, their performance approaches (and sometimes exceeds) that of the twenty-year-olds with whom they are often compared in these laboratory tests.

The memory experiments show other important things. Older subjects do proportionally much better when they are encouraged, not threatened, and when the memory test they are given does not require them to learn and remember something very fast.[21] In other words, if we are frightened and convinced we are doing a poor job, our memories will be worse. We concentrate on our fear and cannot focus on what we want to learn. Being under time pressure adds to the anxiety, and because of the decline in thinking speed it may be impossible for us to store or retrieve the information we want to remember. Finally, the studies show that particularly as we get older, hints or cues to stimulate remembering help tremendously. It is much better to know that a restaurant's name begins with A than to know nothing at all.

Improving Your Memory

How can you use these facts to help you have a better memory? Let's first consider the basics, then look at specific memory-enhancing techniques.

If you are genuinely concerned about your memory, visit your doctor and have a checkup to reassure yourself you do not have a brain condition such as Alzheimer's disease. Treatable illnesses, dietary deficiencies, or side effects of medication, which your doctor can diagnose, may also be making your memory worse. *If you are alarmed by forgetting that seems far beyond the trivial, bypass your family doctor and visit a center specializing in the diagnosis of memory disorders* (see chap. 9).

Next, be aware that the same essential for keeping intellectually fit applies to that special facet of intelligence, memory: keeping mentally stimulated. If you have a chronic condition, guard against excess disabilities; keep as mentally active as possible. Before using any of the following techniques, make sure your life is interesting—that is, memorable. We cannot have a good memory if we have no reason to remember things.

Finally, try to evaluate whether your memory has indeed gotten much worse. Since you have no objective guidelines, this critical question will be difficult to answer. But you can get some idea by asking yourself these questions: "Do I get most upset about my memory when I am feeling down in the dumps?" "Is my inability to connect faces with names really so different from my ability in the past?" "Can I honestly say I never used to forget appointments or my keys to the extent I do now?" "Am I depressed?" (see the next chapter). If you have considered these possibilities and are still convinced that your memory is poor and are truly bothered by your tendency to forget, read on.

MEMORY-ENHANCING TECHNIQUES

First, list the specific memory difficulties that upset you most (e.g., forgetting names). Getting what we want to remember into long-term memory demands focusing. We are incapable of focusing on everything at the same time. Concentrate initially on improving just one of the things on your list, the problem that is most troublesome to you. This will make success possible, and later you can expand what you have learned to other areas.

The research suggests as an older person you have to manage the time you spend on memorizing and recall with particular care. Try to avoid any pressure to do things quickly. Give yourself plenty of time to practice the following memorization techniques. When you are under pressure to remember something not quickly available to consciousness, try to stall. For instance, if you must come up with the name of a person or a book, say graciously: "Didn't I meet you at so-and-so's party? Wasn't our hostess great?" or "I loved that book about dogs. I thought you were someone who would share my taste."

Don't be so nervous about remembering that you ensure your mind will go blank. Try to regain some perspective when you feel your anxiety level rising. Forgetting things happens frequently to everyone, even those who call their memory good. If you can understand this book, your mental powers must be acute!

Another difficulty is likely to be concentration. You must be aroused enough emotionally to focus on what you want to remember, but not so anxious that you can't listen at all. Don't daydream while reading a book and then wonder why you can't remember the plot. Read while you are awake and alert. If your mind begins to wander, decide "I'm too sleepy or preoccupied; now may not be the right time to read." Don't worry so much about remembering the name of the person you are being introduced to that you become certain to forget.

Remembering names and what is read (or heard) are memory problems older people typically complain of. So let's outline how, by devoting real effort, you can make your ability in each area not just better but excellent.[22] But first, let's look at a way to minimize another type of forgetting, the memory problem closest to my own heart—remembering where my elusive purse could possibly be.[23]

Remembering the locations of items. The way to remember where to find objects like your purse, glasses, or keys entails not so much a memory-enhancing exercise as a way of restructuring your life. When we regularly misplace items, the problem is not memory but organization. If we had a definite place for each thing, we would be unlikely ever to forget where it is.

The solution is to select a place for each item and make it a habit always to take the few extra seconds to return objects to their proper places. Having a defined location for items like dishes or socks is something most of us have been trained to do. But not many of us have a firm location for those unique, essential items that are in even more constant use—reading glasses, purses, and such. If, as is true for me, frantic room-to-room searches for a missing purse have already robbed you of weeks of productive life, it's time to establish definite places for these items too.

Unless you live in a small apartment where one location will suffice, designate two places in your house "priority-object sites." Your locations should be widely separated, chosen so it is never too much bother to reach one or the other from any place you tend to put down those important, easily misplaced items (for instance, a table by the door and your night table). Get into the habit of always putting items such as your glasses or purse or keys in one of these places.

Use the same strategy when you are away from home. For instance, decide that "by the door" will be your priority-object place when visiting a friend or staying in a hotel. At a restaurant or a meeting, use the area underneath or beside your chair. If you are right-handed, use the area to the right of you. If you are left-handed, use the area to your left.

The next strategies, because they involve actively exercising your mind, do require sustained effort. But if you master them you will have a great advantage in life—the tools for excellent recall in a wide variety of situations.

Remembering names. Let's say you are introduced to someone at a party and want to remember the name should you ever meet again. To ingrain it firmly in long-term memory, you need to do two things: repeat the name as often as possible, and make it absolutely unforgettable by associating it vividly with the face of the person it belongs to.

Step 1: Repeating. When you first meet, make sure you hear the person's name clearly. Many people, when introducing someone, mumble or slur the name. If you do not hear initially—which is not unlikely in a noisy place—there will be nothing to recall or forget. Say something like: "Sorry, I didn't get that name" or "Would you please spell that?" (You might ask the person to repeat the name even if you did hear it, since this will give you a chance to hear it again.)

Next, talk to your new acquaintance for a few minutes and use the name as often as possible in your conversation: "So nice to meet you, Mr. Johnson"; "Do you live in Manhattan, Mrs. Mahoney?" "I agree, Mr. Smith." If repeating the name like this seems awkward to you, it probably won't to the other person; it is more likely to seem flattering. To me, someone who uses my name often when we talk seems particularly sincere and involved. About four repetitions should give you adequate time to accomplish your next step, making the name meaningful by using the memory aid called association.

Step 2: Associating. Associating is generally helpful in remembering any name, whether of a restaurant, a play, or a person. It involves making what you want to recall stick in your mind by using your imagination to create a picture—that is, a visual image—linking the name with the person, place, or thing. Let's look at how you can use association to remember your party acquaintance's name.

As you are talking, be thinking about how the name could mean something definite—anything concrete that can be pictured with the face. Once you have found your way of giving the name meaning, form a visual picture including it and the person. Don't worry if your image is unusual or bizarre. The stranger the image, the more effortlessly it will float before your eyes the next time you meet the person.

For names that already evoke objects, places, emotions, or anything specific, this task will be easy. For instance, Mrs. Rose could be imagined standing in a garden of roses. Mr. Barber could be seen cutting someone's hair. Miss Paris could be pictured next to the Eiffel Tower. But as shown below, with ingenuity and imagination the same approach can be used with any name. You just have to change its sound slightly or be content to focus on only part of the word in forming your picture.

Here's how I would use association to remember the names of three people I interviewed for this chapter—Silverstein,

Lawton, and Adler. You can practice by trying to come up with different concrete meanings and visual associations for these same names.

The name Silverstein includes the meaningful words *silver* and *stein*, so I would use them to form my image. I might picture Mrs. Silverstein sitting with several bags of silver and holding a stein of beer; or using just the first part of her name, I might imagine her with flowing silvery hair. In either case, the next time I saw her, the bizarre picture I had constructed would reappear. Once I remembered the image it would be easy to recall the name.

I would use the same technique with the other names, Lawton and Adler. Here, though, I would have to be a bit more imaginative to get my concrete images. I might picture Mrs. Lawton in a judge's robe dispensing a severe sentence—*law* (the judge) plus *ton* (heavy or severe). I could change the name Adler to adder and then imagine Mrs. Adler with a huge calculator or holding a long list of figures.

It also helps if you can associate the name with some aspect of the person's appearance such as facial features, mood, or dress. Does Mrs. Silverstein dress expensively? (Is a good deal of silver needed to clothe her?) Does she have beautiful silvery hair? Is Mrs. Adler always looking addled (upset)? How a person looks presents many possibilities to hang your association on.

Use the same approach in remembering other types of names. To recall the name of a restaurant, the street your friend lives on, the title of a book or movie: (1) clearly notice or attend to the name; (2) repeat it as often as possible; and (3) associate it in a picture with a feature of the place or thing. Books, plays, movies, restaurants, even streets are sometimes assigned names based directly on their focal point (e.g., the restaurant the Palm Court; the popular medical thriller *Coma*; the street River Road), so they can be even easier to remember than the names of people or animals.

Remembering story lines or plots. This technique is helpful in recalling any "story," whether it is a book, the nightly news, a movie, or a lecture you just heard.

To illustrate, let's imagine you want to remember a chapter

in a book—perhaps the very chapter you are reading now. Your memory task is to recall the first half of this chapter in unusual detail. Because they already are emotionally charged, you are likely to effortlessly recall the few facts I have presented that are especially relevant to your life. Remembering practically everything in order, though, demands special work. Here are the steps by which you will be able to perform this considerable feat of memory.

Step 1: *Reduce the material to a manageable number of main points and list them.* Encapsulating the content into an outline of six to twelve important ideas will vastly reduce the amount of material you must remember. Once you have the cues provided by memorizing your list, you will be able to ''remember'' or embellish on what the ideas mean and so have almost perfect recall.

Step 2: *Make each idea as personally meaningful as possible.* Ask yourself how points one, two, three, and so on apply to your life. Have you had particular experiences related to what I have said? Do you have emotional reactions to my points? Best of all, use the principle that forming an image helps. Can you get a picture in your mind illustrating each idea from something that has happened (or could happen) to you? Here is the way the first part of this chapter might be reduced to main points and each point made salient emotionally.

1. ''Older people are often anxious about their memories.'' Is this true for me? I remember that last week when we were together, my friend Jane confessed she worries about her memory all the time.
2. ''Everyone—including older people—misreads normal forgetting in a person over sixty-five as a sign of mental confusion.'' It's annoying that people my own age are their own worst enemies. Sometimes I make this mistake too.
3. ''Older people are not good judges of their memories.'' I'd better think about depression, not that big D, dementia, the next time I worry for days about forgetting an appointment.
4. ''How does getting older affect our mental abilities?'' I

wondered about that yesterday when my grandson ran logical circles around me in the political discussion we had.

5. "It used to be thought that intelligence begins to decline early on. Now we know this is not true; older people are unfairly handicapped when taking IQ tests." How terrible that we were so unfairly judged! I can just imagine myself in a room taking the test next to my grandson. Me with my fifty-year-old eighth-grade education, he with his Ph.D.!

6. "IQ tests measure book learning, not real-world intelligence." That explains why my friend's genius son has been such a failure all these years.

7. "Tests of real-world intelligence will measure how we think about real-world dilemmas, not how well we produce academic facts." That seems reasonable to me. That type of test would be just my meat!

8. "What does the standard IQ test tell us?" I'm interested in that too.

9. "As we get older, crystallized intelligence—our sum total of knowledge—tends to increase." I can remember the word *crystallized* by thinking of a diamond, impervious to destruction and increasing in worth as the years pass.

10. "As we get older fluid intelligence—our ability to analyze new information quickly—decreases." I can remember the word "fluid" by thinking of rapids coursing over a dam, rushing by and soon gone. It's true I don't think as quickly as I used to.

I packed a good deal of information into the first pages of this chapter. This dense content has now been reduced to a manageable ten statements. Memorizing this not overwhelming list has been made easier because each thought is now "memorable"—either by being made vivid through an image or by its personal relevance. Anyone doing this exercise can stop here. But particularly if the plot you are memorizing (unlike that of this chapter) must be learned in order, it may help to go one step further. You should have a method of getting easily from idea one to two to three. To make the transition from idea to idea easy, use this approach.

Write down a question that flows logically from the first idea and automatically takes you to the next. True, the linking questions you come up with also will have to be learned. But here your memory job will not be too hard. Each statement you have already remembered should naturally imply the linking question. The linking question in turn will be "answered" by the next idea in the chain. Here are some linking questions I might construct to get from main point one to point three.

Statement 1, "Older people are often anxious about their memories," would be followed by the linking word "Why?" This would enable me to remember point 2: "(Because) everyone, including older people, misreads normal forgetting in a person over sixty-five as a sign of mental confusion." A logical next transition question might be, "But will I really know if I am mentally confused?" The answer here is statement 3: "Older people are not good judges of their memories."

As practice, see if you can make up linking questions to connect the other seven main points above. I think you will find it intellectually stimulating, though admittedly it is very hard work. Then check to see if the technique really is effective by testing yourself one week from now. You may be surprised at how much information you have retained.

As long as you are fully awake, it is best to do a memory exercise of this type in the evening. It is easier to remember something if sleep prevents it from being immediately followed by competing information.

Don't be intimidated by the effort involved in constructing a long list, then making up linking questions, then committing everything to memory. I am just illustrating how it is possible to have, if not photographic recall, then recall that is almost exact. Knowing something this thoroughly is really not necessary, so this technique can normally be greatly simplified. To remember the gist of any story more than adequately, construct a few main points, link them with a few connecting thoughts, and generally see how the plot applies to you.

The main features of these strategies can be used to improve your memory in practically any area. To help yourself memorize anything better: (1) make an effort to focus or concentrate on it fully; (2) make it vivid or important personally—visualizing it in an arresting image helps; and (3) if you have to commit a good deal of information to memory, reduce the mass of material to a manageable set of main points or more general categories. Constructing general categories, for instance, is helpful if you want to recall a long list of items. For example, to remember a grocery list, categorize foods as meats, dairy products, and so forth.

The Shortcut to a Better Memory: External Aids

Unless becoming a mental Hercules is your goal, it is silly to force your memory to do everything on its own. Entering the grocery store with a written list is much saner than burdening your mind with the heroic task of remembering everything you need. Keeping an appointment book is far preferable to memorizing your dinner date for two Tuesdays from now. So anyone who is upset about forgetting should rely heavily on helpers such as the written word. Here are some common things we forget and some creative ways to enhance your memory by external aids.

Problem: Remembering to turn off the stove, remove the laundry from the washer or dryer, or leave the house on time for an appointment. *Solution:* Use a kitchen timer. Set it for the appropriate time and take it around the house with you to be sure you hear it.

Problem: Remembering to pack all the clothing (and other items) you need for a trip. *Solution:* Do not put items into the suitcase randomly. Make a list of what you want to take. Start with shoes and work upwards to hats. Cross off each item as you pack it.

Problem: Remembering to remove food from the freezer. *Solution:* Hang a note on the freezer door the minute you decide what you want to cook.

Problem: Remembering to take essentials such as keys or purse when you leave the house. *Solution:* Pin a note to the door. Have you forgotten your keys? Did you remember your purse?

Problem: Remembering whether you took your medication.

Solution: Every Sunday before you go to bed, put out the next week's medication. Cut up an egg carton or buy a pillbox and put each day's pills in their own space. Then checking whether the space has the pill you are concerned about will tell you what you want to know. (The previous chapter has a more detailed set of strategies for remembering your medication.)

Problem: Remembering birthdays or anniversaries. *Solution:* At the beginning of each month, mentally go through children, grandchildren, and close friends. Ask yourself who is having a birthday or an anniversary that month. Then write down the month's list and post it where it is easily seen. Make it a habit to look at the list every Sunday night.

Problem: Remembering what you came into a room to get or do. *Solution:* Do the chore the second you think about it. Or write it down to do later.

A good deal of effort can be saved by using your mental powers mainly to come up with creative props rather than memorizing everything. But for those of you who are determined to be heroic and develop your memory muscles, there is this final advice. Once you have mastered your projects or reached your goals, if you are truly serious about making permanent improvement, *continue to exercise!* One of the discouraging things researchers observe is that older people learn new memorization strategies easily and well. They can indeed help dramatically. But as with any project that takes work, people often backslide. So keep using those new techniques and extending your memory skills to new things. And remember the essential message (or true gist) of this chapter. It is not true that as we get older our minds dull or our memories must begin to go. What we do can make a big difference in how we think.

For More Information

Hobson, J. "*PT* Conversation with Marian Diamond, A Love Affair with the Brain." *Psychology Today* 18 (1984): 62.
A researcher who has done studies showing that our brain changes physiologically when we are in a stimulating environment dis-

cusses her fascinating findings and explains what her research implies.

United States Department of Health and Human Services, Public Health Service. *Medicine for the Layman: The Brain in Aging and Dementia.* NIH publication 83-2625. Rockville, Md.: National Institutes of Health, 1983.

Clearly written summary of what we know about mental change and the physical changes in the brain that occur in normal aging versus dementia. Write to Clinical Center Office of Clinical Reports and Inquiries, Building 10, National Institutes of Health, Bethesda, Maryland 20892 for copies.

MEMORY-ENHANCING BOOKS

Furst, B. *Stop Forgetting. Expanded by L. Furst and G. Storm.* Garden City, N.Y.: Doubleday, 1972.

Strategies for developing a better memory.

West, R. *Memory Fitness over Forty.* Gainesville, Fla.: Triad, 1985.

Excellent book on memory in middle and later life written by a leading memory researcher. Includes information on how to diagnose any memory loss as well as a wealth of specific memory-improvement techniques.

(For recent memory-enhancing books, check your local bookstore.)

CHAPTER

3

PERSONALITY

My mother was always a vital, energetic woman, but her energy in the last decade of her life took another form: always complaining about minor aches and pains; traveling from doctor to doctor for advice about imaginary physical complaints. Her absorption in my father and us was transferred to an obsession with herself. She stopped growing mentally. She lost interest in new ideas. I'm afraid that now as I'm reaching my seventies, this transformation will be my fate too. Will I get boring, rigid, neurotic, and self-centered, as it seems so many people do? Please don't let me lose the joy in living that seems to evaporate the longer we live. Give me the sense to know if I am becoming the complaining, disagreeable person my mother was toward the end. Is what happened to her normal? Can I do anything to stop it from happening to me?

Built into our thinking are two contradictory ideas about how getting old changes us as people. These harsh black-and-white feelings may be a residue from childhood. Children see their parents and other "old people" ambivalently, both as very wise and also as foolish—stodgy, backward, rigid, and behind the times. Which thought we most believe as grownups may have a good deal to do with our personal experience, how the people we are closest to really do change as they grow old.

Unfortunately, this woman saw her mother change for the worse. So she agrees with the widespread idea that as we get older we contract emotionally. For her the stereotype that older people are rigid, selfish, foolish, unhappy, and absorbed in the past is true, because she saw this change happen firsthand.

For those of us who had (or have) loving, zestful, interesting parents and grandparents, getting older is more likely to symbolize emotional growth, an idea summed up by the lovely phrase "a mature human being." A mature person has the balanced perspective on living that seems to come about only through having lived. The idea that years of living are necessary to becoming a mature human being was spelled out not by Freud, but by his most famous student, Carl Jung.

Jung's personality theory offers us a positive view of how we change emotionally as the years pass. We wouldn't be happy to leave our thirties if we believed only in Freud's ideas. Freud did consider the essence of mental health to be the ability to see the world as it really is, which implies that emotional growth should happen mainly through years of living. But he also believed our personality is completely set by age five. After this early time, he did not think that our experiences alone, no matter how important, could basically alter us. Without psychoanalysis, he said, we are doomed to deal with stress and life in the same way. Furthermore, he implied that by middle age we enter an emotional decline. He warned his students not to do analysis with people over forty, because by this time they become too set in their ways ever to change their essential character.

Jung, once Freud's protégé, took violent exception. He did not see how everything we are could be laid down by the tender age of five. He believed we have the chance of becoming truly mature people only at the age when Freud thought we were emotionally over the hill—forty or so. Jung and Freud fought bitterly over just this question, and Jung left to develop a view of personality that stresses the ultimate importance of the second half of life.

It was Jung who proposed the idea of the midlife crisis, made a household word in the 1970s by Gail Sheehy's popular book *Passages*. He begins his discussion with the time of life from puberty to about the mid-thirties. During this period, which he calls "youth," but which we would call young adulthood, our life thrust is to establish ourselves. Emotions and drives run high—to satisfy our sexuality, to become successful. We are self-absorbed, obsessed with personal achievement, because we must carve out our niche in the world.

According to Jung, midlife (about 35 to 40) is a turning point. We now are settled. We know the shape of our capacities, the contours of what we can do. We either are successful or are beginning to make peace with the idea of not setting the universe aflame. We can stop being absorbed with self-advancement and start advancing as human beings. If things go right, there is a transformation in our personality. We become more mellow and introspective, less concerned with our status and ourselves. We become mature human beings.

Negotiating this transition is hazardous. We are doomed to be unhappy if we "carry the psychology of the youthful phase" into middle and later life. If we remain immersed in narcissism, continuing to lust after applause, we will grow bitter and rigid when the clapping inevitably dies down as the years advance. According to Jung, "We cannot live the afternoon of life according to the programme of life's morning; for what was great in the morning will be little in the evening; and what in the morning was true in the evening will become a lie." A great beauty of twenty can be arresting at sixty too, but only by changing her focus, from her outer to her inner self.[1]

Jung believed that making this change completes us as human beings. Our personality is balanced. We can accept and express every facet of who we are. One aspect of this fuller expression is a loosening of the rigid sex roles that are so sharply defined when we are young. As women get older they are freer about expressing the assertive, "masculine" side of their personalities. Men are more comfortable being sensitive and nurturing, aspects of their inner selves they earlier would have denied and shunned.

Does this starry-eyed view of what *can* happen come to pass, or do most of us stay the same or become more rigid and bitter as the years advance?

Men, Women, and Maturity

Contrary to what the media tell us, the much-talked-about midlife crisis rarely occurs, at least in the heart-wrenching way it is supposed to. Few of us move to Tahiti or violently reject everything we have done in the past forty years. Nor do we suddenly leap to maturity when our hair grows gray. But keeping in mind that we are talking about averages and subtle shifts, some research suggests that in many areas Jung may be surprisingly right.

In about our late thirties, our feelings about time tend to change. From thinking of our future as limitless, we begin to think of life in terms of years left to live. Our goals and aspirations are rearranged. We begin to make more realistic life plans based on a new, more accurate worldview.

Psychologist Bernice Neugarten discovered this change more than a quarter-century ago by looking at business executives in their mid-thirties.[2] About a decade earlier, Neugarten and her University of Chicago colleagues had launched research on personality and aging by doing a different, much larger-scale study.[3] In search of answers to that fascinating question, "How do we change emotionally as we grow older?" they chose a group of "typical" Americans, about seven hundred white, middle-class men and women ranging in age from forty to ninety, in a typical American city (Kansas City, Missouri). For the next six years, they plumbed their subjects' personalities and feelings, examining how they lived their lives. They found that by later middle age, a psychological transformation was indeed taking place.

Jung's prediction was being borne out. The sexes were becoming very similar in personality; they were even trading traditional roles. The older women were more dominant and assertive, the older men more gentle and submissive, less interested in power, comfortable taking a more subservient role. These people were studied before the women's movement, before the emergence of the thirty-year-old female business executive, the new, nurturant young man. But research done in the 1970s at the height of the women's movement, using sources as different as dreams, personality tests, and the positive feeling about leaving work that most men have at retirement's brink,[4] suggests that men and women may become more similar emotionally (or even reverse sex roles) in the second half of adult life.

The shift is also reflected in folklore and myths. The tough, cruel old woman is a common figure in children's fairy tales from around the world; so is the gentle, tenderhearted old man. On the other hand, many leading personality researchers do not agree that this change does take place.[5]

David Gutmann, director of the Older Adult Clinic at Northwestern University, has devoted his career to arguing the pro side of the debate. At the International Congress on Gerontology in 1985 he reaffirmed his views:[6] The personality differences between the sexes have not changed with the sexual revolution, he says, because they are built into our nature as human beings. Women are biologically programmed to want to nurture and men to want to conquer during the first half of adulthood because of the requirements of raising children. Young children should (ideally) have one parent who aggressively provides for their physical needs and one parent who looks after them emotionally, who offers the traditionally feminine qualities of understanding, patience, and selflessness. Once our children are adults, though, we do develop more balanced personalities because we no longer have to follow the biological rules that nature has built in to help ensure the growth of our young.

Recently Gutmann and Northwestern University psychologist Kathryn Cooper found support for the idea that caring for children dampens a woman's assertive drives and accentuates her "feminine" self. They compared a group of women in their forties with children still in the house with another group the identical age in the "empty-nest" phase of parenthood. As they predicted, the empty-nest women were more assertive, less passive, and more likely to describe themselves as "masculine" than the women still immersed in raising a child.[7]

Older people I interviewed for this book describe having changed much as Gutmann describes. Women frequently tell me that over the years they have become less docile and subservient; men say age has mellowed them, made them more interested in the "real" values—family and relationships. But couching these changes just as less "masculinity" or "femininity" seems narrow and negative. The transformation may be part of a larger, very positive picture. I feel that as we grow older many of us become more self-confident, freer to allow our "real selves" to come out.

Now is the best time of my life. What other age offers us such freedom to be self-indulgent and let our true selves flower? My interest in the arts and in helping people was formed early on. But the depression put the luxury of expressing myself through work on permanent hold. Though I never really thought about it until these past few years, I think I was unhappy all of my working life. My job in the garment center was the complete opposite of who I really am. I am soft-spoken, am interested in culture, and consider being a gentleman one of the goals to which human beings should aspire. Seventh Avenue is ugly, filthy, and thumbs its nose at every gentlemanly grace. From the vantage point of my liberation I can't get over how well I survived in that cutthroat job for thirty years. I so easily became expert at the frantic push to get on the packed subway and the routine, mandatory business lie: "You should get that shipment next week; we just sent it out." (Never mind that we had a flood in the factory and that the goods we promised are ruined.) I also can't believe how easily my personality could change over twenty-four hours. I was soft-spoken and gentle at night, tough and abrasive by day, never talking if I could yell. No, I don't feel we basically change as we get older or reach sixty-five. But who we are can look distorted at any time of life when we have to make compromises and adjust to reality in order to live.

When women become more self-confident, they may outwardly appear—and inwardly think of themselves—as more "masculine." In truth, they are just as womanly but have shed the negative trappings of the feminine role: taking second place, avoiding conflict, censoring their true thoughts.

One of the greatest thrills of being a woman of seventy is having the luxury to be open about what I really think. When I was younger, I was so afraid of hurting people or worried about what they would think of me that I rarely criticized; I kept my mouth shut. Now when I don't like something, I speak up. It's gotten me into trouble with my daughter and sister, but I don't care. It's not that I try to be mean, or faultfinding, or unpleasant. It's just that age has made me more truthful. And that's one of the reasons that I feel better about myself now than I have at any other time in life.

These people are more content now than ever. Aren't happy people like them a minority after sixty-five? Luckily the answer is no. They are much more typical than we have been led to believe. Though the media tell us older people are miserable, surveys show that Americans over sixty-five are *not* more unhappy or more depressed than the rest of us. In fact, recent studies done not just in America but in other countries suggest that, if anything, the elderly have lower rates of dissatisfaction and psychological distress than adults of any other age.[8] A nationwide poll conducted by Louis Harris in 1981 had the same theme. One-third of people over sixty-five agreed with the statement, "Now is the *best* time of my life."

A glance at how this large national sample of respondents answered other life-satisfaction questions on the Harris poll shows that there are plenty of unhappy older people, just as there are plenty of unhappy people of any age (see table 2). But getting older does seem to make us less troubled in at least one important way. Emotional problems characterized by anxiety—phobias, disabling fears—are relatively common among children and young adults, but epidemiological (population) surveys show that they are not nearly as prevalent among middle-aged and older adults.[9]

It may be that the most anxious people tend to die off relatively young—for instance, succumbing to stress-induced middle-age heart attacks. People who survive to old age may be emotionally (not just physically) tougher. Or Jung may be right: as we get older we really do mellow. Experience with life's punches may help us react more philosophically, particularly when a major crisis occurs.

The Baltimore Longitudinal Study of Aging, sponsored by the National Institute on Aging, described in chapter 1, is bearing out Jung's point of view. The psychologists in the multidisciplinary NIA research team have been examining how volunteers of different ages react to stressful events.[10] They find that most people of any age do respond in a mature way to life's blows, using strategies such as acting rationally, thinking positively, or crying on a close friend's shoulder to

Table 2   Life-Satisfaction Questions from the Harris Poll

Question	Yes (%)	No (%)	Not Sure (%)
As I look back on my life, I am fairly well satisfied.	87	11	2
Things I do are as interesting to me as they ever were.	69	27	4
As I grow older, things seem better than I thought they would be.	53	38	9
I expect some interesting and pleasant things to happen to me in the future.	62	28	11
I am just as happy as when I was younger.	48	48	4
I feel old and somewhat tired.	45	51	3
This is the dreariest time of my life.	27	70	3
Most of the things I do are boring or monotonous.	21	76	3

Source: *Aging in the Eighties: America in Transition* (Washington, D.C.: National Council on the Aging, 1981).

Note: People over sixty-five were asked whether they agreed with the statements.

help them cope as constructively as possible. But mature reactions are most common in middle-aged and older people. The volunteers aged twenty to forty-nine were more likely to handle setbacks badly—flying into a rage, escaping into fantasy—than those aged fifty to eighty-nine.[11]

And the Baltimore study is proving Freud wrong. As we grow older, we do not get more rigid. We are just as flexible as ever in dealing with life's changing demands. When they analyzed the ways volunteers dealt with stress as they returned over the years, the psychologists found: "Older men and women do not rigidly maintain habits of coping that . . . have outlived their usefulness. Instead, as stresses change so do coping responses."[12] Or—put more bluntly—we mature dogs are just as able as ever to learn new tricks.

Other research shows we may be particularly good at coping with life's most devastating traumas. The myth is that the elderly are least able to handle the worst. If anything, the opposite seems true. For instance, of any group, *elderly* women are least apt to develop severe physical or emotional problems after a spouse dies. (In chap. 7 I will offer a possible reason for this fascinating typical finding of the widowhood research.)

Being older also seems to make it easier to handle a life-threatening disease. When researchers at the University of Southern California studied 369 patients newly diagnosed with breast, colorectal, or lung cancer, they found that the age of the victim made the biggest psychological difference. Older people handled the shock of the news better; they were psychologically stronger in facing the disease.[13]

Emotional hardiness is not confined to people with advantages like money or high social class. In a large study of stress among working-class elderly people in North Carolina, six months after having even several major setbacks, most people showed no serious psychological effects.

I am not suggesting that we should calmly shrug off traumatic events. After getting a diagnosis of cancer or losing a loved one, it may actually be healthy to feel bereft. Some psychologists believe that people who put a lid on their feelings and go on just as normal after such tragic events suffer worse pain later on. (Once again, see the chapter on widowhood for a more complete discussion.) But there are also dangers in prescribing how anyone should behave. There may be no rigid "best" way to handle life's worst blows, because a variety of methods work. By "work," I mean they help us to function and go on living, not necessarily that they ever totally erase our pain. And depending on who you are, you will handle problems in your own distinctive way.

The Ways We Do Not Change

Is our distinctive way of dealing with problems fixed too? Freud may be wrong about our becoming more rigid, but isn't he right about our essential character? Aren't we basically the same people at seventy as we were at twenty-five?

The answer is a qualified yes; we can see many seeds of that old person in the youth on the brink of life. National Institute on Aging psychologist Paul Costa and his colleagues have marshaled compelling evidence that our personalities remain remarkably stable over large chunks of adult life by examining how the personality test scores of Baltimore study volunteers change as they return over the years. Costa finds that getting older does not bring more conservatism, or more self-absorption, or more immersion in the past. The best prediction about how the years will change us is that they will not.[14]

Costa's research shows that certain broad aspects of personality are quite stable throughout adult life: introversion versus extraversion (Do you love going out and meeting new people, or do you often feel more comfortable being alone?); cautiousness versus openness to new things (Do you adore new experiences, or are you uneasy deviating from the tried and true?); and unfortunately, the tendency to be emotionally disturbed. People who are extremely depressed, hostile, anxious, and poorly adjusted in their twenties and thirties are likely to have emotional problems in middle and old age.

These findings refer to our inner dispositions, not necessarily to how our actions appear. So the many of us who describe ourselves as shy may look extraverted to our friends or even say we have grown out of our shyness as the years advance. But we don't turn into real extraverts, because we still have a flutter of anxiety before going to a party. We can't get over those ordinary people on the street who can open their mouths and say something coherent when the camera zooms in for the nightly news. These events are feats for us. Shyness—or severe emotional problems, or reluctance to try new things—is a part of our personality we fight against, sometimes well, but tend never to fully conquer.

Many of us would agree with Freud in blaming our parents, feeling that during our childhood they taught us these fears that now keep us from fully enjoying life. We would be partly wrong. Psychologists now think that genetics, not upbringing, can have a significant effect even on such surprising aspects of who we are as our gestures, the people we like best, or our moral values. Just as we inherit the shape of eyes and face, we are born with different temperaments that determine the general outlines of our behavior. And by comparing adopted children with their biological and adoptive parents and looking at the personalities of identical twins raised together and apart, researchers have shown that the tendency to be shy or to have severe psychological problems is indeed somewhat hereditary. It's not that we are fated to be introverted or schizophrenic by our genetic makeup. It may be that a loving environment can still go a long way toward changing the negative predispositions we have. It's just that seeing Mom and Dad as the cause of every deficiency isn't fair either.

These facts do not bring encouragement to people who believe that getting a job, or winning the lottery, or living more years will bring happiness. Happiness is not determined by what happens to us. Optimists find happiness in a dungeon; pessimists see sadness in the most heavenly life. In his most recent research (involving a national sample of thousands of men and women), Costa and his coworkers find that growing older may mute the intensity of our highs and lows (we may become less emotional as the years pass); but it has absolutely no effect on overall happiness.[15] Happy thirty-year-olds are likely to be happy at eighty—though at eighty, thirty-year-old joie de vivre looks more like quiet contentment.

But Costa is looking at averages and so, as with any view of the whole forest, he misses some interesting trees. Even he admits the clarity of the crystal ball varies from person to person. While most people may not change in some very basic ways as the years advance, some of us change a good deal. Who are the people who change the most? More important, who is likely to ripen or wither emotionally as they grow old?

Two Keys to Ripening with Age

In the early 1970s Henry Maas and Joseph Kuypers offered some clues when they restudied a group of middle-class people who had been interviewed and tested forty years earlier in a depression-era study of child rearing.[16] The University of California researchers had information about these people as young parents in their thirties. What would they be like in their seventies?

In agreement with Costa, Maas and Kuypers found that the people who had genuine emotional problems in their thirties had changed little. They were still hanging on by their toenails to life at seventy, as they had been at thirty-five. Some of the more emotionally stable majority changed a good deal. People changed most when their outside lives had become most different; that is, when a good deal had happened to them over the years.[17] For instance, if you are a widow and have had to go to work for the first time, you are likely to change more than your friend who is still married and whose life, except for the children's being grown, has stayed about the same. If you are not debilitated by illness, though, one influence seems particularly important in whether you are likely to grow or decline emotionally as the years pass: Does your life fulfill your inner interests and capacities?

Maas and Kuypers found that if a woman's only interest in her thirties had been her husband and children, she was more likely to be unhappy in later life. Some people who had chafed at being just wives and mothers were more fulfilled in their seventies because for the first time they found what fit them. They had never liked the housewife role. At seventy they were finally able to live as they wanted—to have a career. And for many lucky people life was good in their thirties and kept getting better. They were happy at any age because they always were able to arrange lives that were fulfilling to them.

A study published much more recently—in 1987—underlines exactly how crucial it is to arrange an outer life that fits us.[18] Rutgers University psychologist Daniel Ogilvie asked a group of retirement-aged men and women to rank their "identities," the life roles that were most meaningful to them (e.g., mother, gardener, choir member, caregiver to ailing mother, highly organized person, pillar of the community). He then asked how much time they actually spent acting out these most meaningful aspects of themselves and probed their morale—how satisfied they were with life. The two assessments were closely related. People who spent the most time living out their highest-ranking identities were the happiest human beings. While we cannot expect perfection, the lesson of this study is that one key to happiness in our later years is to spend as much time as we can in meaningful activities, enacting life roles that genuinely express our inner selves.

After leaving high school I went to work as a bookkeeper because of a bad experience. I had a disturbed teacher and was afraid if I got a degree in education I might turn out like her. Now I know I would have loved teaching because of my joy in running this group.

God has given me the chance for a second life at my advanced age of seventy-nine. Since my heart attack and bypass surgery two years ago, I feel even more in awe about this "extra" time on earth.

But I really came into my own in my late twenties, when I married a wonderful man. My parents objected. He was a plumber—not our social class. They came around. I did the bookkeeping for his business. I tried for years to get pregnant and then had my one beautiful girl. Until his death in 1969 of cancer, Max and I were ideal partners. When bad things happened, we stuck together. Because we could bob up after the worst problems, we called ourselves the two corks. I was almost suicidal for several years after he died. But then, six years ago, I got this chance at a job I feel I was almost born for. At a discussion group at our synagogue, the rabbi asked if one of us would want to start a senior citizens' group. Money was there for a painting teacher and speakers, and there were some rooms we could use. When nobody volunteered, to my astonishment I said I would. I think it was my horror at the idea that the money would go somewhere else!

It was hard at the beginning, but I kept going because of my daughter. She always said, "You can do it," as I moaned about how silly it was at my age to take on something this scary and new. Now that things are running smoothly, I know taking the risk was the best thing I've ever done. Planning our activities, speakers, and trips fits in so well with my training as an organizer working with Max. I love being close friend, educator, surrogate mother (and boss) to our more than ninety regular members. Most important is the sense of satisfaction. People come feeling lonely and at loose ends. Some have had strokes or are very depressed. Our group makes a difference in their lives. It has done everything for mine!

Because of a lucky opportunity in her seventies, this woman was able to find the perfect "job," one that drew on all her skills and allowed her talents and interests to flower. Life does not often dish up such a perfect chance for self-fulfillment. It is even less likely, as was true for this woman, to be almost forced on us in later life. But she had the strength to accept when her chance came rather than giving in to the idea that an older person shouldn't try something new. In part this was because she had the support of her daughter, a second ingredient that the research suggests promotes happiness in later life.

People who care about us push us to take risks that are emotionally hard. They also are a buffer against life's blows. While this is true at sixteen or at sixty-five, the importance of close, supportive relationships for older people in particular has been repeatedly demonstrated in studies done over the past twenty years.

In the late 1960s Margery Fiske Lowenthal of the University of California surveyed the frequency of psychological problems among all the residents over age sixty in a low-income area of San Francisco. More than anything else, she found that having a "confidant" (someone to confide in) helped these people bounce back emotionally after the most devastating tragedies rather than breaking down.[19] This compelling evidence of the importance of having at least one close relationship was followed by an avalanche of studies tracing the effect of what social scientists call "social support" in cushioning stress. As it turns out, not only do close relationships help us weather life's slings and arrows, they even reduce our chances of getting physically ill.

For instance, in the Alameda County study (discussed in chap. 1) researchers have found that social isolation is a significant risk factor for earlier than normal disability and death. In this ongoing research, thousands of residents of Alameda County, California, are being followed to see the effect of health practices (e.g., exercising, not smoking) and social factors (e.g., living an isolated life) on longevity. According to George Kaplan, who reported on the study's results as of 1986, being married has virtually no effect on life expectancy, but having at least one close relationship does. Older people who have a confidant tend to live longer than those who do not.[20]

As we get older and our loved ones die, our store of confidants erodes. But if the ranks of your friends have thinned, do not despair. It is the quality, not the quantity, that counts. The studies show that older people with many living relatives, many neighbors, and many "social contacts" per day or week are no happier or more protected from stress than anyone else.[21] Being surrounded by critical or uncaring people may even be worse than having no one at all. Are other people important to our health and well-being? Yes, *provided they are genuine confidants*—supportive, understanding, caring presences.

What the Studies Mean to You

The research shows that rigidity, boredom, and increased self-absorption are not natural to growing old. They are as much signs of a problem at eighty as they are at eighteen. So is unhappiness. Particularly if you were happy and well adjusted earlier, you are set up for happiness after age sixty-five. But you can get derailed. The danger of becoming bitter and unhappy is greater if you do not have at least one close relationship; it is predictable if your current life does not fulfill you and help further you as a human being. Unless you are very ill (when we are sick it is hard not to be depressed or self-absorbed), these impediments to happiness can be changed.

A major problem is giving up, becoming immobilized by the idea that because you are older you should put your personality on hold: "Now that I am sixty-five, the time for living fully is over. I should be staring into the sunset or sitting in a rocking chair contemplating the fire. At my age, withdrawing from the mainstream of life is right." The idea that doing nothing is right at any age is wrong. Doing nothing is tailor made to produce unhappiness. Depression is a natural consequence of sitting and staring at a wall.

Helplessness, Control, and Growing Older

Psychologists believe that when healthy older people just retire to a rocking chair it is because they have a problem. They may be suffering from a condition called "learned helplessness.'' Learned helplessness comes about when, after losses, failures, or being treated as incompetent, we lose faith in our ability to do *anything* effectively. This lesson in the futility of action profoundly affects our emotions and the way we behave. We become apathetic, withdrawn, and hopeless about the possibility of ever finding pleasure in life.

Parents can easily produce learned helplessness in children by punishing them often for no reason. This gives them the idea that they are helpless, that anything they do is ineffective or wrong. We can also develop this debilitating problem at any time of life when misfortunes wash over us and it seems we have lost the power to control what happens to us. But because uncontrollable losses do occur more frequently and the options to act can seem less, the danger of developing learned helplessness seems greater after retirement age. The subtle insinuations that age brings incompetence also take their toll.

I am continually surprised at how even people only ten years younger than I am see an active, obviously healthy older woman like myself as a doddering idiot. They speak more loudly, assuming a hearing problem I don't have. They talk more simply, assuming I am on the verge of Alzheimer's disease. They treat me more gently but discount what I say and do. I wonder how often people my age relax and come to agree—giving in to these expectations and giving up.

Judith Rodin of Yale University has studied the corrosive effect of being helpless not just on our psyches, but on our bodies too. With Harvard psychologist Ellen Langer, she selected a group of nursing-home patients and gave them a few more responsibilities and choices. Could they care for plants in their rooms? Could they choose the menu for that day? Nursing-home residents are physically dependent. Their lives are externally regulated to an extreme. As the ultimate helplessness-producing environment, the researchers felt a nursing home would be an ideal laboratory for studying the life-enhancing effect of being a more autonomous human being.[22]

Adding just this dollop more of autonomy had a widespread impact. The residents perked up, becoming more alert and feeling happier. The change was long lasting, still there at an eighteen-month follow-up. And the intervention affected not just the quality of life, but its length. Whereas the overall mortality rate in the home was 25 percent, over that period only 15 percent of the residents who were given more autonomy and responsibility died.

At the 1986 meeting of the American Psychological Association, Rodin summarized the growing body of research demonstrating that having control over one's life and being given more decision-making power increases longevity in the elderly.[23] She urged caution too. The studies have been done with nursing-home patients. They may not apply so well to the much greater autonomy of noninstitutional life. And having more responsibility is not right for everyone. Some of us are uncomfortable making decisions. We want other people to take over; we are happy to have the anxiety inherent in making choices removed. Or more likely, we want to be able to make our own decisions about A, B, and C but want others to take over X, Y, and Z. Assuming control where we don't want it can boomerang, making us anxious, perhaps even shortening our lives. So exercising choice and being master of our fates is important, but so is selecting the level of control and decision making that fits us.

Here is a classic instance where having full decision-making power could cause added emotional distress: Your doctor brings up the possibility of surgery to correct your son's birth defect. The procedure has the potential to severely exacerbate his condition or to cure it. After carefully spelling out the risks of surgery, your physician leaves the choice totally up to you. Would you feel less anxious if Dr. Jones simply took control, saying, "In my professional opinion, Joe should have this operation"? In this situation many of us might opt for less control. But how can you tell if you are suffering from the opposite problem—not enough say over your life? The best way is to examine the symptoms that learned helplessness produces. We know these symptoms by another name—depression.

Are You Depressed?

The emotional problem of depression is not the same thing as the sadness, frustration, and unhappiness we all feel occasionally as the price of being alive. It is a real mental disorder that can have a number of causes. Learned helplessness is just one. Genetics, early life experiences, personality, current and past losses and failures, and overwhelming stress all may produce or contribute jointly to a person's becoming depressed. Although the symptoms and severity of the illness can vary greatly between individuals, if you are depressed you will experience one and probably several of these changes.[24]

Marked, long-lasting mood change. Have you been gloomy, sad, and unhappy for *some time?* Are you neglecting your grooming? Are other people regularly reading unhappiness in your face and posture?

Change in appetite. Have you lost interest in food? Have you lost weight without trying? (Loss of appetite is a more typical sign of depression than overeating.)

Sleep disturbance. Are you having regular problems in falling asleep? Do you often wake up early (at 3:00 or 4:00 A.M.) unable to get back to sleep? (Understand, however, that some lessening of the time we sleep is normal in later life.)

Changes in thinking speed and activity level. Are you constantly agitated or unable to sit still? Do you feel jittery most of the time? Or are your body and mind operating in slow motion? Are you unable to think clearly or move quickly?

Inability to experience pleasure. Are you preoccupied with thoughts of doom, dread, or foreboding? Have you lost interest in everything? Are you always tired, lethargic, and apathetic?

No depressed person has all these symptoms. You can even be depressed without feeling sad. Sometimes lack of appetite, or insomnia, or vague physical complaints are the only symptoms, and a depressed person runs from doctor to doctor in search of an elusive disease. Or cloudy thinking may be the main sign and so an older depressed person is mistakenly diagnosed as having Alzheimer's disease. So diagnosing depression can be difficult; even a trained observer may be fooled.

GETTING TREATMENT

If you persistently have any of these symptoms, have a physical checkup. Fatigue, problems in eating or concentrating, and weight loss are also signs of most diseases. Depression is a common accompaniment of hypothyroidism, Addison's disease, Cushing's disease, pernicious anemia, idiopathic parkinsonism, uremia, congestive heart failure. It is associated with cancer of the pancreas, leukemia, and brain tumors; it is a side effect of a variety of drugs (see table 3). Rule out any medical reason for your symptoms first.

Then ask your doctor to recommend a mental health professional—a licensed psychiatrist (M.D.), clinical psychologist (Ph.D.), or clinical social worker (M.S.W.).

Or visit your local community mental health center (look in the Yellow Pages or inquire at your local hospital), which offers treatment on a sliding fee scale. Particularly at clinics where students are being trained, the quality of services can be top-notch, because people are learning the most up-to-date treatment techniques.

According to various community surveys, anywhere from 5 percent to 50 percent of older people suffer from depression. Gerald Klerman, professor of psychiatry at Massachusetts General Hospital and an authority on the subject, estimates that less than one-quarter of the older people who are depressed get any treatment at all. Cloudy thinking, fatigue, lethargy, problems in eating and sleeping—even chronic unhappiness—are too easily passed off as normal old age, particularly in a person whose worldview is gloom and doom. Many people think that if they seek out psychological help they must be crazy. Or they may realize they have an emotional problem yet not go for treatment because they (rightly) recoil at endlessly, expensively, and embarrassingly discussing what happened fifty years ago.

This is unfortunate. According to Klerman, "treatment of depressions and other affective disorders is often a gratifying experience for patients and their families. Because of the range of biological and psychological treatments that are available, patient response is generally good." Depending on the cause of your depression, medication alone may be effective, or you may need medication plus psychotherapy, or psychotherapy alone.

Psychotherapy is most effective for the type of depression that is triggered by an external—that is, situational—cause. You've never been the same since the death of your wife; since developing your disability, you feel apathetic and hopeless

Table 3   Some Medications That May Produce Depression

Class and Generic Name	Trade Name
Antihypertensives	
Reserpine	Serpasil, Sandril
Methyldopa	Aldomet
Propranolol hydrochloride	Inderal
Guanethidine sulfate	Ismelin
Hydralazine	Apresoline
Clonidine hydrochloride	Catapres
Antiparkinsonian	
Levodopa	Dopar, Larodopa
Levodopa and carbidopa	Sinemet
Amantadine hydrochloride	Symmetrel
Hormones	
Estrogen	Femestral
Progesterone	Lipo-Lutin, Progestasert, Proluton
Corticosteroid	
Cortisone acetate	Cortistab, Cortelan
Antituberculosis	
Cycloserine	Seromycin
Anticancer	
Vincristine sulfate	Oncovin
Vinblastine sulfate hydrate	Velban

Note: Consult your doctor, since this list may not cover newly developed drugs.

about life. Sometimes the reason people become depressed is genuinely physical—a defect in brain chemistry is producing symptoms that often seem to arise "out of the blue." For these "biological" depressions, drug therapy is the treatment of choice.

The newest form of psychotherapy for depression has much more in common with taking a course than with being on the couch. You are taught strategies to control your depressive thoughts and helped to take action. You and the therapist collaborate (more as teacher and student than as doctor and patient) to identify the "helpless and hopeless" ideas that are preventing you from getting pleasure from life and take concrete steps to change your life so you feel more fulfilled.

This treatment, called cognitive behavior therapy, is effective. Research presented by Stanford University psychologist Dolores Gallagher at the 1986 meeting of the American Psychological Association showed that a twenty-session treatment regimen totally cured or greatly improved about 70 percent of a group of depressed elderly patients. The effects were long lasting. Most remained symptom free or had only minor symptoms at a one-year follow-up.[25]

If you have a mild case of learned helplessness, let's see how you might use a cognitive behavioral approach, plus the information in this chapter, to find a more fulfilling life. (Unfortunately, people who are suffering from learned helplessness to any real extent are by definition incapable of helping themselves. They desperately need professional help to change their conviction that they are helpless and that their situation is hopeless.)

Finding More Fulfillment

RETRAINING YOUR THINKING

Use the research to school yourself in a new way of thinking about "old age." The personality changes called "natural" to getting older are far from natural at any age. Being bored or self-absorbed or unhappy has nothing to do with being over sixty-five.

Monitor your negative thoughts. Each time you think "A person of my age has to be bored," catch yourself: "I'm unhappy not because I'm seventy-five, but because right now I'm not doing anything that grabs me emotionally." Stop thinking "Depression is the price of living to eighty" and label your mental state for what it is: "I am dissatisfied now because of X, Y, and Z in my life." The advantage of this new way of thinking is that it stops you from throwing up your hands. If what bothers you is in your situation and not basic to you, you can do something about making a change.

It should be obvious from this chapter that this new perspective is accurate. Being sixty-five or eighty-five is far from tantamount to having an unhappy life. Older people are not less happy. Many say they prefer now to any other time of life. Getting older may lessen our anxiety; it seems to strengthen us emotionally in facing stress. Take advantage of the inner strength you have accumulated in years of living to utilize the opportunities for personal growth that are out there for you. Search out the fulfilling experiences that are so necessary to feeling happy and involved at any time of life.

Understand that you do have options. If you are in the grip of learned helplessness, this may mean changing another ingrained idea: "Nothing exists for a person my age. What I can do is severely limited. There is little chance of having a life that expresses my inner self." This way of thinking is also untrue.

There is a widespread idea that the world offers few meaningful opportunities to older people, perhaps because important identities through which we *have* found meaning, such as "raising my children," are indeed gone. But there are replacements, new identities that can be developed, new ways of getting satisfaction from life. As we get older, what expands is the potential for expressing oneself as a person apart from the traditional roles of "mother" or "breadwinner." A whole new set of choices opens up because the old roles that took all our energy are over (or less all encompassing). Some of these choices are age restricted. They become possible only after age sixty or sixty-five (or fifty).

The Epilogue of this book is devoted to exploring some new options that open up after age sixty or so—the special educational and creative opportunities specifically for retirees or older people; how to find fulfillment as a volunteer; how to look for a paying job. Chapter 8 describes new living arrangements such as retirement communities. Read this information now if you cannot shake the feeling that nothing is out there for a person past late middle age.

Don't cut yourself off from opportunities for "senior citizens" or "retirees" because they conjure up images of doddering people in wheelchairs. You'll be surprised at the effort devoted to self-enhancement, the high quality of what is going on, and the interesting people who are not inhibited about taking advantage of what is newly available once society defines them as "senior citizens." Considering that today "senior citizen" is a label likely to apply to people for twenty years or more, it far from means waiting in the wings for death.

Systematically analyze your life. After reframing your attitudes, you need to decide what specific directions to pursue. Drawing on the research on "identities" discussed earlier, begin by getting an overall sense of how well your current life fits your inner self. List your most meaningful roles, your prized traits and skills, and the aspects of yourself you value most (e.g., musician, good cook, giving person, organizer). Assess how much time you actually spend enacting these most meaningful identities. Then devise specific strategies to increase this time. "I think I could devote at least five more hours a week to my music if I did X, Y, and Z." "If I invited guests for dinner at the house each Sunday, I could really indulge that most adored activity in my life—preparing gourmet meals." "That volunteer job helping the homeless find shelter and negotiate the system seems tailor-made to satisfy my need to give to others and draw on my talents as an organizer."

If your list of current meaningful identities seems meager, this is a signal that you need to construct new compelling roles. Evaluate your present life. Are there interests, activities, new roles you haven't attempted but think you might enjoy? What has stopped you from trying these new things—inertia, fear, your feeling that chance just isn't out there? Would you prefer to do something new where meeting people is likely, or don't you care about that?

Although you certainly can develop totally new identities, the research also shows that in many ways we don't change that much. The things you used to enjoy doing are the things you are most likely to enjoy now. So if you are unsure what could have meaning, think about what has had meaning before. Carefully explore your past. Imagine yourself in your teens, your twenties, your thirties, and so on. What special interests consumed you? Are there aspirations you have always wanted to fulfill? What were your talents or skills, your greatest pleasures? Are there things you have always wanted to do but never got the chance to try? What barriers prevented you from doing them then? Would the same inhibitions or external difficulties keep you from fulfilling these dreams now?

Remembering what used to interest you is helpful if you go blank when thinking about anything that could give you pleasure now. If every new possibility makes you yawn or just seems too hard, forcing yourself to do something that used to excite you can sometimes prime the emotional pump. When we begin by going through the motions of doing something that used to thrill us but that we can't imagine enjoying now, an emotional connection is sometimes remade. Almost magically, the good feeling starts flowing again.

Even if you are sure what directions you want to pursue, this exercise may be revealing. It is easy to overlook other things you might enjoy. Reviewing your life also helps you plan realistically, by getting you to pinpoint your lifelong strengths and weaknesses, the things you know you can do or would be too frightened to do. Because these aspects of personality are also likely to stay the same, they should be respected, or we may be doomed to fail in attempting anything new. Your job is to make the difficult task of constructing new identities as easy as possible emotionally and to use any strategy that has been helpful to you in the past to get you going in arranging a more fulfilling life.

Get confidants involved in your plan. Take into consideration the other point the research makes: having someone who supports you will help. If you have good friends, feel free to lean on them. Don't listen to well-meaning loved ones who tell you it is inappropriate to go back to school, or work, or "exert" yourself at your age. If loneliness and isolation are important problems for you, choose something new that involves meeting people who could be potential confidants. Concentrate your search on places and activities where you have a good chance of making friendships. Many opportunities for "retirees" or "senior citizens" have a built-in social component. People participate both because they want to do new things and because they are looking for a more socially enriching life.

TAKING ACTION

Set a deadline to stop thinking. Get a large calendar and mark a date to take action.

Break carrying out your plan into small steps and make a timetable for completing each. "The first week in July I'll call the volunteer bureau; week two, go for an interview; by the end of July (I hope) start." "This summer I'll rent a place in that retirement community I'm considering moving to; if I like it, I'll put my house on the market in the fall. My deadline for making a permanent move will be a year from now." The important thing is to keep to your plan and reward yourself generously for every step forward. Post your calendar in an eye-catching place, a testament to whether you are fulfilling your goal.

Enlist a buddy if possible. Another prod to get yourself going is to undertake your new activity with someone else. Going somewhere with a buddy makes it emotionally easier and also forces us to take action, something that is hard for many of us to do. To some extent we are all cautious (rather than thrilled by the idea of new experiences). What psychologists call "the shy gene" is commoner than we think. It may even be built into our nature as human beings. But given that new beginnings and entrances are so hard, when we don't have the comforting physical presence of a buddy, is there anything else that will help ease the way?

Try to find a supportive friend or relative whom you can regularly tell about your progress, who will be present in spirit as a buddy. Inform her about your plan and the schedule you have made. Check in at predetermined times to tell her if you have followed each step. Have her praise you lavishly for success but gently push you to meet your deadlines. This is the technique that has made national organizations like Alcoholics Anonymous and Weight Watchers so successful. You can use the same principles on your own to engineer a more satisfying life.

You don't even need a buddy. Use the same strategy toward yourself. Reward yourself with some special treat (e.g., those earrings, those theater tickets, that delicious meal cooked just for yourself) for major advances toward your goal. When you have reached your goal, celebrate.

Evaluate your situation after two months. Once you have started, don't be afraid if you don't like what you are doing at first. Give yourself two months or so of going through the motions before you decide whether you chose correctly or were wrong. It often takes some time before the anxiety subsides and we connect psychologically. It is a rare person who fully enjoys anything new in the first few days or weeks. Keep remembering that you went into the activity with your eyes open. But if you still don't feel happy beyond, let's say, the two-month cutoff date, don't hang on expecting things to magically change. Decide to cut your losses and leave.

Don't give up and return to doing nothing if your first choice isn't satisfying. To get some perspective (and decide what else you might want to try), once again review your life. How often in your past has that first job, or first relationship, or first anything been the one that worked out in the end? One great advantage of having *many* experiences is that they give us a broader perspective on the importance of individual failures. The ability to have this less emotional, more realistic view of single things that go wrong is what Jung probably meant by our needing to live life to become fully mature.

For More Information

Jung, C. J. "The Stages of Life," trans. R. F. C. Hull. In *The Portable Jung*, ed. Joseph Campbell. New York: Viking, 1971.
   Jung's theory of life's stages.
Rodin, J. "Aging and Health: Effects of the Sense of Control." *Science* 233(1986):1271–76.
   Excellent, though difficult, article summarizing the research on helplessness and health in the elderly.
Seligman, M. *Helplessness: On Depression, Development and Death.* San Francisco: W. H. Freeman, 1975.
   The learned-helplessness theory explained in depth.

PART

II

RELATIONSHIPS

4

LOVE, MARRIAGE, AND SEX

My first husband died when I was thirty-five. For the next eighteen years I focused my energy on working and raising my children. I rarely dated and had no sex at all. I felt my sex life was over. I had had passionate sex with John. It was unlikely that at my age I would ever find anyone else.

When I was fifty-three, I met a man ten years older than I was. We fell in love. The thrill is just as powerful as with my first marriage. If anything, maturity has added a new dimension and depth to what was there before. My marriage, now twenty years old, is very happy—sexually and in every other way. Murray is over eighty, but he is still able to have intercourse. Our sex is less frequent but in some ways better because it is more relaxed. At our age love means companionship: doing things together, communicating. Our marriage does not live or die depending on his erection on a particular night. Being older has made us more secure. We are not afraid of being honest. We tell each other how we want to be touched. We are satisfied physically when our lovemaking does not end in orgasm. We are more tolerant and tender both in and out of bed. I want young people to know. Marriage is better after retirement, when the children are gone; this is the time of life when experience and leisure peak and we become able to give fully to a husband or wife.

Does marriage grow better as the years pass? When sociologists at Miami University of Ohio reviewed a variety of studies of marital happiness, one-third bleakly confirmed the old jokes: happiness peaks at the honeymoon, and over the years it steadily declines.[1] Familiarity and the pressures of child rearing lead to disenchantment. By the twentieth anniversary, what was there is either disintegrating or gone. And people never recoup what is lost. Couples stay locked in disenchantment after their children grow up and they are alone together again.

But half of the studies showed there is truth to the idea of a second honeymoon. Marital satisfaction dips dramatically after the children are born, reaching its lowest ebb during the turbulent years when a middle-aged couple has adolescents in the house. But it rises again after the nest is empty. We can regain what we once had when we are free from the pressures of bringing up children and have the luxury of focusing on one another again.

For instance, Robert Atchley and Sheila Miller found long-lived marital happiness in full bloom among a large group of mainly white, middle-class, elderly couples.[2] The Miami University researchers interviewed their subjects—residents of a pleasant midwestern community—periodically from 1975 to 1981 seeking answers to these questions: How do upheavals such as retirement, changes in health, or a recent move (being a new arrival in the town) affect a marriage? How similar in values, interests, and goals are husbands and wives who have been married for decades?

Neither retirement nor moving affected the high degree of marital happiness that was typical. And these long-married husbands and wives were amazingly alike; on a long list of goals and favorite activities, they gave identical answers an average four-fifths of the time. The people married longest were most similar, giving scientific weight to the cliché, "When they've been together that long, they even begin to look alike."

The researchers loved doing this study, saying, "It was a genuine pleasure to be around these couples. They accepted one another fully, were obviously devoted to one another, and were very much enjoying their lives together."

Poor health was the only cloud in these sunny marriages. If a husband or wife became sick, the partner's happiness tended to take a nose dive. The men were most vulnerable; they seemed more dependent on their wives than vice versa, because having a healthy spouse was absolutely central to their marital happiness.

It makes sense that illness would shake a happy marriage. It is hard to be giving when your energy is consumed by aches and pains. It is hard to enjoy your marriage when your job suddenly shifts from life companion to nurse. And when illness strikes an older couple, the nursing job does fall hard on the well person's shoulders, even when there are grown children around. Studies agree, when a husband or wife is alive, sons and daughters tend to shy away from really stepping in. It is all the more remarkable, then, that even in the midst of the upheaval, many elderly couples do regroup, close ranks, and stay firmly committed to each other.

Even the most distressing illnesses can draw a couple closer. For instance, when researchers probed the emotions of husbands caring for wives with dementia, one-fourth of the men said their wives' illness actually heightened their feelings of closeness and intensified their feelings of love.[3] Being thrust full time into the role of caregiver takes away from friends and other activities, making the marriage the total center of life. And when the possibility of losing a loved one looms close, what we have is transformed from a given to a gift. What may have been taken for granted for decades becomes precious and irreplaceable. Illness tugs strongly at our sense of obligation, too.

In the early 1980s University of California anthropologist Colleen Johnson interviewed elderly couples after either the husband or the wife had been discharged from a Bay Area hospital.[4] She probed the feelings of both spouses separately, asking these middle- and working-class older people about the quality of their marriages, the amount of conflict they had, how emotionally fulfilling the relationship was. Only one-quarter said they had any major disagreements; most felt they could firmly rely on their husbands or wives for emotional support. These people were obviously taking seriously their vows of in sickness or in health.

The only chink Johnson found was the unemotional, stoic way husbands and wives described their marriages: "We've survived fifty-five years of it. Today they only last two or three years." "He's been a good provider and a good father." "Long ago I realized you can't change horses in midstream." True, these couples were content; but passion was just as obviously gone.

Johnson feels that in later life good marriages should be judged by different criteria. As the years pass we may be cemented not so much by the intensity of our emotions as by the length of our history—our backlog of shared ups and downs. "The fact of a marriage's mere survival connotes success."

These studies show that marital happiness is alive and well among elderly couples. But if I had described others, a much less upbeat portrait would emerge. Distance, disappointment, and isolation blight many long-lasting marriages too, especially among the very old.[5] So while knowing that older couples can be happy—and often are—is encouraging, the obvious truth is that marriages differ greatly, in old age and at any other age. Can they be classified?

Different Types of Marriages

In one study, long-term middle-class marriages fit into three general types, two unhappy and one ideal.[6] In the "conflict-habituated" marriage, quarreling and nagging were the main forms of communication. Husbands and wives were locked into a protracted undeclared war, but neither seemed interested in divorce. It was as if each person derived a perverse pleasure from having someone to fight with.

The second kind of marriage was the one the researchers found most often—the passive/congenial relationship. This marriage was less stormy but just as unfulfilling, lurching along indifferently and joylessly. Husbands and wives stayed together physically but remained separate emotionally. They had marriages of convenience without understanding or love.

I have nothing in common with my husband. We can spend the whole evening together—he and I staring at the TV—and I couldn't think of one word to say to him even if you paid me a million dollars. My husband is a good provider. I would not think of getting a divorce. But emotionally there is nothing

*there—no real love or closeness. After forty years of marriage
he lacks any interest in me or understanding of who I am.*

The third kind of marriage is one we all want or may be
lucky enough to have, "the vital relationship." As the researchers described it: "The vital pair can be easily over-
looked. . . . They do the same things, publicly at least and
when talking. . . . They say the same things—they are proud
of their homes, love their children, gripe about their jobs. . . .
But when we take a close, intimate look, the vital quality of
the relationship becomes clear; the mates are intensely bound
together psychologically in important life matters. Their sharing and togetherness are genuine. The relationship provides
the life essence for both man and woman."

WHAT IS YOUR CHANCE
OF HAVING A VITAL MARRIAGE?

Robert Atchley and Sheila Miller's study, discussed earlier,
implies that one key to a vital marriage is having the externals
in place. Their happy Ohio couples had enough money, had
good health, and were living in a close-knit, crime-free community. Clues to what will happen later also may be apparent
early on. People who are delighted with one another after
years of marriage say they were always very happy with their
mates.[7] On the other hand, starting out a marriage without
love or loving less than fully is a bad sign; although love can
deepen over the years, rarely does something grow from absolutely nothing.

*It's my fiftieth wedding anniversary, and I'm bitter. I am mar-
ried to a person who shares none of my interests. My husband
is an alcoholic loudmouth. Can't tell him anything. He is
stubborn and flares into a rage at the least little thing. He loves
me—or says he does—but I do not love him. I never have, and
how I wish I really knew what love is! You see, I got married
out of need at a low point in my life. I was in a car accident
that left me partially paralyzed, feeling terribly unlovable and
sorry for myself, and he was the first man who came along.*

As a fascinating 1987 research report shows, perhaps the most important clue lies in one's personality and the personality of one's spouse. Lowell Kelly of the University of Michigan and James Conley of Wesleyan University studied several hundred married couples over a forty-five-year period, tracing their lives from their engagement in 1935 through 1980.[8]

Twenty-two couples broke their engagements, and fifty got divorced over the years. Another group stayed unhappily married, together by default. Of the many factors the investigators examined—stressful events during the marriage, education, occupation—these failed relationships were distinguished more by the psychological instability of their participants than by anything else. A man rated as emotionally disturbed at the time of his engagement was likely to have marital problems. A neurotic new bride was set up for an unhappy marriage or a future divorce.

Whether a couple stayed together and was miserable or got divorced after years of marriage turned out to be a function of the *man's* personality. Neurotic men with low "impulse control"—those who acted out their misery—were prone to engage in behavior (such as having affairs) that would force an unhappy union to end. If a man was neurotic but high in impulse control, he did not act on his unhappiness, and so the couple tended to stay married. In other words, in depression-era marriages, at least, the man holds sway over the union's fate. Not only do his actions initiate a marriage, they terminate it.

Elderly New Lovers and New Marrieds

So far I have been discussing what happens many years later to people who walk down the aisle at the typical age. What is love like when it strikes in our autumn years? To answer this question, sociologists Kristine and Richard Bulcroft used the membership list of a Minneapolis–Saint Paul singles club to find a group of autumn lovers, people ranging in age from sixty to ninety who were romantically involved but not married.[9] They interviewed these elderly lovers, comparing their responses with those of college students in love.

Being older did not dim the heady symptoms of romance. The older lovers felt the same heightened sense of reality, awkwardness, heart palpitations, intense excitement, and sweaty palms as the twenty-year-olds. As one sixty-eight-year-old divorcée said, "When you fall in love at my age there's initially a kind of 'oh, gee!' feeling—and it's just a little scary."

Nor did age weaken the lure of the trappings of romance. Both young and elderly lovers enjoyed candlelit dinners, long walks, flowers and candy. The older men agreed with the young men about the most romantic shared activity it was possible to have. As one seventy-year-old put it, "You can talk about candlelight dinners and sitting in front of the fireplace, but I still think the most romantic thing I've ever done is to go to bed with her."

There were differences, too. Among the older lovers the involvement was faster paced. People said that at their age there "was not much time for playing the field." The older people were also more realistic about those heady first sensations. Most had been in marriages that had lasted decades. They knew their racing hearts would quiet down and understood the value of what they hoped would follow—a more long-lasting love that grows out of knowledge, out of appreciating a real human being.

Yeah, passion is nice—it's the frosting on the cake. But it's her personality that's really important. The first time I was in love it was only the excitement that mattered, but now it's the friendship—the ways we spend our time together—that counts.

Luckily, in this study the idea that older lovers have to fight disapproving children was not borne out. When the relationship was made public, most sons and daughters accepted or welcomed it. Some would invite Mom or Dad's date to family get-togethers or to dinner at their homes. But the women particularly were often uncomfortable about letting their children know, sometimes devising elaborate strategies to conceal what was going on—hiding a lover's clothes when the grandchildren came over, bringing along the cordless phone on the nights spent "at his house."

There were other difficulties in having an autumn rather than a spring romance. Unlike the younger lovers, the older people had more trouble deciding whether having sex was right; although the rules today have changed, they grew up with a system of values that said extramarital intercourse is always wrong. In spite of their awkwardness, most decided yes. Sexual involvement tended to develop early and was usually a vital part of the relationship. While couples enjoyed intercourse, they valued other aspects of sexuality just as much—kissing, caressing, cuddling. As one seventy-seven-year-old woman said, "Sex isn't as important when you are older, but in a way you need it more."

Few of these people wanted to get married. The women were especially reluctant, reasoning that making things legal was unnecessary. They did not have the push young people have to make a family or a life together. They also were afraid a trip to the altar would mean being saddled with the vow "in sickness or in health." Many had nursed a husband for months during his final illness. They did not relish the thought of more years spent as nurse to a sick spouse. (As we will see in the chapter on widowhood, this emotion is shared by a surprising number of older women.)

To find out what happens when people do take the plunge, marrying a second time after age sixty-five, sociologists at the University of Evansville interviewed a group of recently remarried older couples.[10] These elderly new marrieds—drawn randomly from Evansville, Indiana, city marriage records—were not younger, better educated, or better off financially than the typical older resident of the city. They *were* dramatically different in health. According to this study, people who get remarried in later life are much less likely to be ill than their contemporaries.

Some of these people remarried soon after being divorced or widowed. But many had lived many years before finding a new mate. The women were most surprised at the turn their lives had taken. Half said they had been sure they would never marry again. Among many reasons given for remarrying, companionship stood out. People married mainly to have someone to travel or do things with; falling in love ranked a distant second. And those female concerns about being a nurse may not be idle fears. The men—not the women—in this study often said they wanted to remarry in part to have someone to take care of them.

These marriages, now all in their second to sixth year, were working out. The couples agreed they were happier than their first ones. They felt their new marriages were better because now they themselves were more mature. And marital happiness came easier at this time of life because the stresses of child rearing and establishing a career were past.

A survey of several thousand Consumers Union subscribers over age fifty also reveals that autumn unions are unusually blissful.[11] Although many of the couples in this large national study were contented, people married less than five years reported the highest conjugal bliss. The only other group that approached them in happiness were the golden anniversary couples. According to this survey, couples who make it to the fifty-year mark tend to be almost as joyous as newlyweds.

Finding out what marriage is like after age fifty was a secondary purpose of the Consumers Union survey. The poll was mainly done to study a more shrouded area of life: sex. Every subscriber to *Consumer Reports* was sent a no-holds-barred, pages-long questionnaire about his or her sexual practices, feelings, and capacities. Respondents voluntarily returned the questionnaires, so those who did participate in this survey are not a random group. They are probably people especially interested in the sexual side of life. Still, the results were a surprise.

Most of us know the idea that sexuality has to die after a certain age is false. But we may feel that getting older means automatically having a much less sexy life. The Consumers Union study showed that this idea is absolutely false. A passionate sex life was flourishing among many of the respondents, including many golden anniversary couples and people with daunting physical impediments to intercourse.

While Kinsey and Masters and Johnson first shed scientific light on our sexual behavior during the 1950s and early 1960s, these pioneering sexologists had little data on sexuality past middle age. Few of their subjects were over fifty. At that time the sexual revolution was just beginning. It was hard to get older people (even men) to mention sex, much less volunteer for a study of it. The Consumers Union poll, two studies done at Duke University in the 1960s and 1970s, and the National Institute on Aging's Baltimore Longitudinal Study of Aging are almost the only large-scale surveys we have of the sex life of older Americans.[12]

There are no rules about what happens sexually as we age. Some people with little interest in sex in their twenties or thirties find passion after fifty, when maturity loosens their inhibitions or fate presents them with the first love of their life. For others passion and performance burn on as strongly at eighty as at eighteen. Without minimizing this diversity, here are some generalizations we can make from these landmark studies and Masters and Johnson's work.[13]

(The information in the rest of this chapter is explicit—designed for people who will not be offended by a graphic description of age changes in sexuality or put off by some very specific advice on lovemaking techniques.)

Male Sexuality

Kinsey and Masters and Johnson found that the frequency of a man's erections and orgasms slowly begins to decline very early, after his late teens. The Duke, Consumers Union, and Baltimore studies show that this regular, decade-by-decade decline continues after age fifty.

The seventies seem to be sexually crucial for many men. In the Duke study, about three-fourths of the men in their sixties were still having intercourse; many indicated their sexual interest was high. But during their seventies most gave up intercourse. The number reporting a high or moderate sex drive also dropped dramatically during these ten years.

The reason seems to be poor health. In their seventies many men began to suffer from diseases. Illness is what tends to greatly dampen a man's libido and his ability to perform.

On the other hand, the seventies are far from a sexual death knell. In the Duke study, half of the men in their eighties had sexual feelings. One-fifth were having intercourse. And even when men (and women) have severe physical problems, they still can have a passionate sex life.

The husband is seventy-six and the wife seventy-four. They recently celebrated their golden wedding anniversary. . . . The husband reports that communications between he [sic] and his wife are very good. . . . Having sexual intercourse together, however, is impossible. Because his wife has a spastic paralysis, she cannot spread her legs. . . . "So," he explains, "we've had to devise an alternative. . . . But it works!" And when occasionally we achieve coincidental orgasms, it's as satisfactory as when we were in our twenties. It's a cooperative effort—a kind of mutually contrived double masturbation." . . . The two have sex together this way about three times a month. She reaches orgasm about 75% of the time, he about half the time. . . . He has enjoyed a variety of sexual activities with his wife since age fifty; undressing her; having her undress him, mutual oral sex, mutual masturbation, manually stimulating her clitoris during sex. . . . He enjoys it when she stimulates his breasts and nipples but he does not stimulate her breasts and nipples because she "had double mastectomy. . . . So this is one activity we both regret we cannot perform." Love as well as sex have survived this husband's erectile problems and his wife's spastic paralysis and double mastectomy. . . . After more than fifty years of marriage . . . he adds "love curve is still upward!"[14]

As long as a man stays interested in sex he can enjoy sex, even with physical problems that rule out normal intercourse. The real fear, though, is not so much losing interest as (put bluntly) no longer being able to "get it up." Realistically, here are the physical changes to expect.

PHYSICAL CHANGES

Erections occur less spontaneously and require more time and effort to develop. In contrast to the twenties, when just seeing an attractive woman would be enough, after fifty a man is more likely to need direct physical stimulation of his penis to become erect. Older men also tend to lose their erections more easily and may get a very full erection only right before they ejaculate. In spite of these changes, penetration is normally not a problem. Impotence is not inevitable to growing old.

The frequency of orgasm lessens. Masters and Johnson

found that most men over sixty need only one or two climaxes per week. This does not mean older men should restrict themselves to once-a-week sex, just that a man who has sex every day or two should not feel upset if he can't always ejaculate. One result of this decreased pressure is a plus from the woman's point of view. Because a man can stay erect longer without having to ejaculate, lovemaking can last longer. And some (but not all) men find that by middle age any youthful problems with premature ejaculation improve.

Ejaculations are less explosive or intense. Not only does the force of the orgasm lessen, the feeling of "ejaculatory inevitability" is lost; older men no longer have the sensation of having to ejaculate several seconds before orgasm.

The ability to have sex right after reaching orgasm is lost. Decade by decade, the "refractory period"—the time after orgasm before another erection is possible—gradually lengthens. Each man's refractory period is different, and its length also varies depending on how intensely arousing a particular sexual encounter is. On average, though, men in their sixties have to wait a day after having a climax to get fully erect again.

These losses can worry people inordinately. After a few instances of failure a man may overgeneralize, jumping to the conclusion that his days as a lover are over. His partner too can overreact: "He must no longer find me sexually appealing." A self-fulfilling prophecy can be set up. Afraid the problem may recur, a couple is tense the next time they have sex. Their anxiety makes a repeat performance more likely. What started as a random incident becomes a fact of life.

How traumatic are performance problems for most elderly men? If we accept what the men in the Baltimore study say, not very traumatic. Among the roughly two-fifths of the men in this study aged sixty-five to seventy-nine who were less than fully potent, only 10 percent had gotten medical help for their condition. Most accepted their problem with relative calm. The researchers hypothesized that the lives of these men were so fulfilling in other ways that sexual performance was not important to their self-esteem.

If you are older and upset by occasional potency problems, Saul Rosenthal, publisher of an excellent newsletter entitled *Sex over Forty,* suggests putting what has happened into perspective. Just because a man of sixty cannot run as fast as he did at twenty does not mean his running days are over. Like any bodily capacity, sexual performance should be expected to change somewhat as the years advance. Changes due to an impersonal process, aging, should not be taken as a personal affront. One instance of "failure" should not be seen as the beginning of the end. After a problem occurs, do not give up having sex, hoping things will improve next month. As with any exercise, the key to staying in shape sexually is to keep active.

There are strong indirect indications that "use it or lose it" are particularly apt words in the sexual realm: the research consistently shows that the best predictor of continued sexual activity in later life is a passionate sex life earlier on.[15] For instance, the most sexually active older men in the Baltimore study did not differ from the other volunteers in education, age at marriage, number of years married, or even marital happiness. They did differ in this way: they had always been very sexually interested and active. A lifelong passion for sex and reasonable good health set the stage for a fulfilling sex life in our later years. But there is another ingredient too—having the flexibility to adjust your lovemaking to aging. Here, from *Sex over Forty*, are some suggestions to help fulfill this important requirement.[16]

ADJUSTING YOUR LOVEMAKING TO AGING

Because erections occur less spontaneously, your partner should manually stimulate your penis; you both should plan to enjoy, not feel threatened by, the age-related slowing down of erection. Enjoy the preliminaries—stroking, touching, kissing. Reorder your priorities. What leads up to intercourse should no longer be viewed as foreplay but as one centerpiece in a total sensuous experience.

Do not set yourself up for disappointment by fantasizing about a day spent in bed making love. Don't give up your plan. Look forward to it in a realistic way. If, after intercourse, you cannot get a second erection, don't get anxious and try to force yourself. Spend the rest of the day enjoying each other's caresses, or try a new sensual activity that does not depend on repeatedly getting erect.

Do not drink too much and then expect to have sex as usual

or have intercourse when you are exhausted or preoccupied. When you were in your twenties your sexual system may have been resilient enough to withstand these stressful conditions. It is more fragile now. Plan your lovemaking for when you feel best. This may mean switching from a routine of sex after the eleven o'clock news to sex at 8:00 A.M., as long as neither you nor your partner has to be at the office by nine. Be able to focus your full attention on one another, not on being tired, or on having to get dressed in fifteen minutes, or on a meeting an hour from now.

Occasional sexual difficulties are normal for almost every man. If a problem occurs during a sexual experience, don't devalue everything. Ask yourself if you enjoyed what did happen. Then explain what you did feel to your partner: "Having an orgasm is great, but it's not everything. I still enjoyed our sex thoroughly."

Keep in mind that a slower erection has its benefits. Women need time to get excited. They don't relish the one-minute-to-orgasm experience that nature forces on many men in their twenties. Take comfort that in middle and later life you may be physiologically more in tune with your lover than ever before. The effects of age on your performance can also force you to be a more sensitive lover. They may push you to be creative, to expand your sexual repertoire from "intercourse as usual" to more varied things (if you have not done so before).

View problems as a challenge, not a defeat. If you are having trouble getting an erection, stimulate your lover to orgasm manually. Get a sex manual. Try lovemaking techniques that do not involve intercourse. If your erection is not fully hard, have your partner lubricate herself with a lovemaking oil to make penetration easier. Massage each other with the oil. Use your problem as a chance to enjoy a new sexual experience. (For erection problems, sex therapists recommend another technique that sometimes primes the pump. The man "stuffs" his limp penis into his partner's vagina. Sometimes the sensation of being in the warm, moist vagina can produce a full erection.)

A relaxed attitude, the ability talk with your partner, and being open to trying new things is crucial. Flexibility, full communication, physical and mental openness are important to having satisfying sex at any age. They become even more critical in later life. Here, from the Consumers Union study, are some testimonials to serve as inspiration. Even severe erection problems need not be a deterrent to a rich, full sex life.

From a retired engineer in his seventies:

> We sleep on twin beds. I fixed one bed so that a pair of footrests can be attached to the foot. . . . My wife can move down so that her hips are right at the end of the bed—with her legs spread apart and resting on the footrests. I get between her legs with my feet on the floor. The height of the bed has been adjusted so she is at the correct height. She is now completely exposed so that I can enter her easily even without an erection [while stimulating his wife manually in this position]. I watch her to judge when she is about ready to have an orgasm, and then make my penetration and we have our orgasms together—which is the ultimate in lovemaking. [Using this technique he adds both he and his wife now aged 74 and 45 each orgasm about 100% of the time].[17]

From a divorcée in her late fifties:

> I sit on his penis and let my partner have his orgasm in my vagina . . . and then my turn comes. With his limp penis still inside me, I rub my clitoris up and down his pubic bone while I enjoy a whole series of orgasms. With this technique, a partner whose penis is limp or who ejaculates prematurely is no problem at all.[18]

IMPOTENCE

It is normal to slow down sexually in later life but still be able to have intercourse. However, some older men suffer from impotence, chronic erection problems that make intercourse impossible. Impotence most often happens when the normal age-related slowing described earlier is compounded by medical conditions that prevent a man from having an erection full enough for intercourse. Among men over sixty, it is estimated that more than 70 percent of the time impotence has a primarily organic cause.

An erection occurs when the intricate web of blood vessels and blood-containing chambers in the penis becomes engorged. The blood flow into and out of the penis is regulated by hormones, nerves, and tiny valves. Any problem that affects the delicate erection mechanism has the potential to cause impotence: disorders affecting the blood vessels (arteriosclerosis, high blood pressure, diabetes); operations done in the pelvic area (bladder, prostate, or rectal surgery); injuries to the pelvic region and spine; diseases such as kidney ailments or multiple sclerosis.

Medications taken for high blood pressure, heart conditions, arteriosclerosis, depression, and anxiety may impair sexual performance. Alcohol is another drug that erodes sexuality. Drinking blocks the erection reflex. Chronic excessive drinking also has a long-term permanent inhibiting effect on sexual capacities because it damages the liver, suppresses the level of the male hormone testosterone, and affects circulation.

The answer to whether a given case of impotence is physical or psychological lies in sleep. Normally men have an erection every ninety minutes during the dreaming stage of sleep, called the REM (rapid eye movement) period. A device attached to the penis and worn for several nights can monitor whether erections do occur during this stage. If they do not occur or occur only partially, a man's impotence has a physical cause.

Great medical advances have recently been made in treating impotence. There are now erection-improving medications. (One muscle relaxant, Papaverine, when injected into the penis, can cause an erection lasting one to two hours). If the problem has to do with the blood vessels regulating blood flow into and out of the penis, surgery on the penile arteries may help keep the penis engorged. And there are devices that artificially support the penis, called penile implants.

Penile implants fit in the penis, producing an erection. There are three types. With the inflatable implant, a man pumps fluid from a reservoir in the abdomen to tubes in the penis when he wants an erection. The semirigid implant produces a permanent erection, one that is less firm than normal but usable for intercourse. Its advantage is that it is more economical and simpler to install than the pump. A third type of implant has been developed that combines the simplicity of the semirigid implant with the realism of the inflatable variety.

None of these treatments is a panacea. They vary in effectiveness, and they may produce complications. Still, depending on the cause of the problem, they may help tremendously.

If sexual difficulties concern you, have your problem diagnosed by a competent specialist—a urologist, an internist, or a psychiatrist who specializes in treating sexual problems. The physician you visit should give you a complete physical; take a careful sexual history; measure testosterone or other hormone levels; test your cholesterol and blood sugar; test for erections during sleep; and analyze whether penile circulation problems are to blame.

If your difficulty is found to have a psychological cause, you may be referred to a nonmedical professional—a psychologist or social worker with special training in treating sexual disorders. The basic principle underlying the psychological treatment of impotence is to reduce the performance anxiety in sexual situations that inhibits an erection. To achieve this goal, couples are often told to take the following steps.

Make love with fingers and tongue but do not have intercourse. If lovemaking does not involve intercourse, then there are no expectations to perform.

When an erection occurs, do not have intercourse. The idea is to practice getting erections easily but keep down the anxiety involved in maintaining an erection for intercourse.

Concentrate on your own pleasure without considering your partner's needs. Because worrying excessively about the other person's feelings tends to inhibit arousal, these instructions help the person's natural responses to emerge.

In addition, a therapist may train a couple in relaxation techniques; teach them to utilize sexual fantasies; give them specific pleasure-enhancing tips. The approach used is tailored to what is likely to be most effective for the particular problem and people involved.

SEX AFTER A HEART ATTACK

A surprisingly frequent precipitant of psychologically induced impotence is a heart attack. After a heart attack, people tend to turn off to sex, afraid that if they get aroused or have intercourse they will have another.[19] In fact this celebrated way to go is highly overrated. In one study of a large group of men with heart conditions who died suddenly, fewer than one-half of one percent died during sex; many more died in their sleep. Eighty percent of postcoronary patients can go back to normal sexual activity a few weeks after a heart attack. The other 20 percent don't have to give up sex totally but can adjust their lovemaking to the level of exercise their hearts can tolerate.[20]

The steamiest sexual encounters are less straining on the heart than they appear. Even the peak pulse rate during the few-second heat of orgasm is likely to be lower than the maximum the average person experiences each day. Walking up stairs, running for the bus, even worrying about personal problems are just as likely as sex to make our hearts race. The physical exertion involved in intercourse is also lower than for many forms of exercise. Walking up two flights of stairs or its equivalent probably puts more strain on the heart than having sex. Here are some tips from *Sex over Forty* for resuming sex comfortably after a heart attack.

You and your sexual partner (who is likely to be just as anxious as you) should discuss with your physician the sexual activities your heart can and cannot tolerate. If your doctor ignores the issue, you bring it up. If he or she seems uncomfortable talking about your fears or gives unsatisfactory answers, get a consultation. Have every concern answered fully, or you will keep worrying and your sex life will suffer.

Learn your exercise tolerance by taking the appropriate medical tests. You might also undergo a physical conditioning program for cardiac patients so your heart will not have to work as hard when you do have sex.

When you resume sex, start slowly, with a week of caressing and petting without having intercourse. This will ease you into lovemaking without your getting too worried. Always take care to have sex under optimal conditions, not when you are very tense or tired.

Experiment with "safer" intercourse positions. Try changing from the man-on-top position to the woman-on-top position (it does take slightly less energy). Try the "spoon position"—you curl up sidewise and enter her from behind. Or if you still are worried about the sex act being too strenuous, make love without having intercourse. Use oral or manual stimulation to bring each other to climax.

Explore medications that may lessen angina. If you have heart pain during intercourse, consult your doctor. Is there a medication to take before having sex?

Avoid sexually impairing medications. Some heart medicines have sexual side effects. If you have lost your sex drive or if having erections becomes noticeably more difficult after the heart attack, ask your doctor if your medication may be to blame. Is there another drug you can take?

Treat depression. Depression, a common reaction to a heart attack, also dampens desire. If you are depressed—an understandable emotion given what has happened—get professional help.

Female Sexuality

Compared with men, women are the physiologically resilient sex. Masters and Johnson found that older women are just as capable of reaching orgasm as young adults. In many areas of arousal and performance, female sexual capacities change little with age.[21] When the years make a woman more self-confident and sharpen her sexual skills, sex may become better after age fifty, more passionate than ever before.

Often this physiological potential is untapped. Although the machinery is intact, the mind turns off. Gaining weight, defining oneself as "dried up" or "menopausal," and putting energy into mothering, not lovemaking, prevent many women from getting to step one—turning the engine on, wanting to have sex.

And it is hard to tango alone. In the Duke studies, "marital status" was the most important predictor of a woman's sex life. Older women with a husband living were likely to still be having intercourse. Only a small fraction of those over sixty who were widowed, single, or divorced were.

While some women are able to stay interested in sex without having a partner—masturbating often, having an active fantasy life—many turn off.[22] Perhaps because feeling desirable is so crucial to feeling desire, while the chance of being without a partner increases as a woman ages, in both the Duke and Consumers Union studies, decade by decade the proportion of women having sexual feelings declined even more steeply than was true for men.

It is also not accurate to say that nothing changes physiologically after age fifty. Menopause does cause physical changes that can sometimes have striking sexual side effects. Fifty is the average age when American women today reach menopause—the programmed shutdown of the ability to conceive and bear children.

WHAT HAPPENS PHYSIOLOGICALLY AT MENOPAUSE?

The monthly cycle of ovulation and menstruation is regulated by hormones secreted by the pituitary and the ovaries. Menopause technically refers to the total cessation of menstrual periods, the end of a woman's capacity to have children. This change is the culmination of an ongoing phase called the climacteric. About fifteen years before menopause, during a woman's late thirties and forties, her reproductive system gradually functions less well. Ovulation and menstruation become increasingly irregular; the chances of miscarrying or bearing a child with a birth defect increase; the ability to get pregnant lessens. This falling off of reproductive capacity and its finale, menopause, are orchestrated largely by a decrease in the female hormone estrogen.

Estrogen depletion has no direct effect on sexual desire; the male hormone testosterone, present in the female body too, regulates the intensity of the sex drive in both women and men. However, it indirectly affects a woman's enjoyment of sex because it dramatically alters the vagina and surrounding tissues, ultimately causing many women discomfort during intercourse. During a woman's childbearing years, the walls of the vagina have thick, cushiony folds that expand easily to admit a penis or accommodate childbirth. After menopause, the vaginal walls thin out and become smoother and more fragile. The vagina also shortens, and its opening narrows. The size of the clitoris and labia decreases. There also is a diminution in the amount of sexual lubrication. It tends to take longer after arousal for a woman to begin lubricating, and fluid is never produced as copiously as before.

Unfortunately, these changes tend to happen at the same time as a woman's partner may be having difficulties with erection. The combination of a drier and less penetrable vagina and a penis less able to penetrate causes some older couples real trouble with intercourse. One method of easing the problem was suggested earlier, using a lubricant—either a lovemaking oil, K-Y jelly, or any substance that makes the vagina less dry. The Kegal exercises recommended to stimulate vaginal tone after childbirth may also help strengthen the vagina. Or relief may be found by a somewhat more controversial route, taking replacement estrogen.

REPLACEMENT ESTROGEN

Estrogen supplements (taken either in pill form or vaginally) lessen many unpleasant postmenopausal symptoms, including painful intercourse. Taken long term beginning at menopause, they are also the most effective treatment for preventing osteoporosis—the postmenopausal bone loss that makes women prone to fractures in later life.[23]

But taking estrogen involves problems. It increases a woman's risk of endometrial cancer (cancer of the lining of the uterus) from about one in one thousand per year to about four in one thousand.[24] It is associated with high blood pressure, blood clots, abnormal vaginal bleeding, and a slightly higher risk of gallbladder disease.

On the other hand, estrogen does not have the frightening side effects that had previously been feared. The latest studies show that estrogen supplements do not increase the risk of breast cancer; they may even help protect against the disease. Taken long term, they may also decrease the chances of a heart attack.

When its link with endometrial cancer was found about a decade ago, many women stopped taking estrogen. Today estrogen supplements are coming back into favor. Not only are the studies of their effectiveness in preventing osteoporosis encouraging this trend, but new research suggests that the risk of endometrial cancer is reduced (or virtually eliminated) when estrogen is given in cycles of three weeks on and one week off and is combined with the hormone progesterone toward the end of a woman's cycle. Also, endometrial cancer is relatively rare in any case, even among women who take estrogen. It is also a slow-growing type of cancer, almost always diagnosed while it can still be cured.

Many experts advise not taking estrogen if you have a family history of endometrial or breast cancer, blood clots, strokes, coronary artery disease, severe migraine headaches, liver disease, or unexplained vaginal bleeding. Before starting, they advocate a thorough medical checkup, including a pelvic examination and Pap smear, breast examination and mammogram, tests for blood sugar, liver and thyroid function, and cholesterol levels. Many also recommend an endometrial biopsy (test for endometrial cancer) as an additional precaution.

For you, do estrogen's benefits outweigh its risks? The Consumers Union consultants recommend, in making a final decision, asking yourself these questions: "Do I need estrogen?" (Am I at high risk for osteoporosis: of small build, a smoker and heavy drinker, sedentary? Are my "change of life" symptoms very upsetting? Is my sex life suffering greatly?) "Do I want to take estrogen despite the risks?"

If your answer is yes, proceed, taking estrogen with progesterone. Get semiannual breast and pelvic exams. Consult your doctor promptly if you have abnormal bleeding. Periodically review new information about estrogen-replacement therapy with your physician.

ADJUSTING YOUR LOVEMAKING TO AGING

Apart from vaginal changes I have just discussed, there are few physiological reasons why getting older should erode a woman's sex life. The studies suggest that the main problem for women is staying interested in sex. Here, from *Sex over Forty*, are some ways to keep desire aflame.

Inject novelty into marital lovemaking. Many long-married women lose interest in making love because they have fallen into a rut. They have intercourse at the same time and place and in the same way year after year. When sexuality becomes predictable, the most fiery passion turns ho-hum. One antidote is to vary the sex act itself. Have intercourse on the floor, in the bath, or in the woods. Experiment with a vibrator. Read erotic literature together. Role play each other's fantasies.

Everything may not work out, but experimenting may help bring back some sexual spice.

Bring back your courtship. Your romance may need rekindling too. Go away for a romantic weekend with your husband. Surprise him with a candlelight dinner, served in a filmy nightgown. *Seduce him!*

Take care of yourself. Keep physically healthy. Exercise. Spend time on how you look. Maintaining sexual desire depends on feeling sexually desirable—taking pride in your appearance, keeping your passion for life. In some ways becoming an older beauty is easier, because as we age how we look is increasingly tied to what we do. While nature has a firm hand at twenty, at fifty nurture (work!) takes over an increasing share. The saying that after forty we get the face and body we deserve has its bright side. If we take action to be attractive, attractive we really can be.

Keep sexually active. If you have no current partner, buy a vibrator. Masturbate; develop a fantasy life. If you have a partner, take the initiative sometimes. Don't always wait passively to be seduced. In their classic studies, Masters and Johnson were surprised to find that the three most sexually active older women they tested produced just as copious amounts of lubrication when aroused as the twenty-year-olds. So they concluded that sexual activity itself may even prevent the physiological losses thought to be inevitable. Staying sexually active seems as much a cure for "losing it" sexually for women as it is for men.

For More Information

Brecher, E. M., and the editors of Consumer Reports Books. *Love, Sex, and Aging.* Boston: Little, Brown, 1984.
 The Consumers Union study, offering statistics on sexual behavior among married, single, and divorced Americans enriched by personal vignettes, information about love and marital happiness, what changes to expect sexually, and advice about how to cope when problems arise. A fascinating book.

Masters, W. H., and V. E. Johnson. *Human Sexual Response.* Boston: Little, Brown, 1966.

Masters and Johnson's classic research on the physical aspects of normal sexuality; also has a chapter on age-related changes in sexual capacity.

Sex over Forty. P.O. Box 1600, Chapel Hill, North Carolina 27515. An excellent monthly newsletter offering sound medical and practical information relevant to almost every age-related sexual concern. To subscribe (or to order back issues of special interest), write to the address given above.

CHAPTER

5

THE GENERATIONS

My family is in California. I love them dearly, but I would rather live here in Chicago. Jack has a heart condition. I have to spend time taking care of him. At age sixty-six I thought I would be free to focus on my number one priority at this time of life—the two of us. If I lived in California, I would never stop running. I would get nervous, resentful, and tired. Everyone would expect all of me full time.

Last year my mother died. My father is in a nursing home. I call his floor every other day to check up. If I lived near Four Oaks I would visit often, crying each time I drove off. It's less painful to imagine him as he was, not have what he has become rubbed in my face—a diminished person, no longer the strong man I adored. My sister Carol, who lives in Beverly Hills, is resentful. She accuses me of dumping the burden of his care on her. Not fair! I am mentally just as involved even if I'm not physically there.

And I'd rather not regularly witness what my forty-year-old unmarried daughter's life must be like. If Karen is as lonely as I fear, I would be too upset. As it is, our long-distance calls don't go smoothly. I can't help asking the off-limits question in the back of my mind: "Are you going out with any men?"

Even Joey and Mark, my daughter Jane's twin boys, are not worth moving for. My exuberant grandchildren are the joy of my life. I take out their pictures, remember the cute things they say, and ache to hug them. But what would it be like to be an on-call unpaid baby-sitter? The temptation to criticize the loose way Jane is raising them would be overwhelming,

*even though the smallest comment makes my daughter see
red.*

*But I must stay half a continent away because of Jack. If I
was always running to my family, he would be enraged. We
planned on this time of life for each other. We were bitterly
wrong. When does the job of family caretaker end?*

Though we might think this woman has many blessings,
the unexpected quality of the woes she is also facing deserves
our sympathy. Within this century, changed demographics
have caused a revolution in family life.

In 1900 most people did not survive past their fifties. If both
sets of parents were alive to dance at their wedding, a bride
and groom felt blessed. Today it is unusual not to see grandparents at a wedding, and even great-grandparents may be
there. Four-generation families are common; five generations
are no longer rare.[1]

In the past, children and parents were grown-ups together
for a short time. Being a grandparent meant delighting in toddlers, if you were lucky enough to see the third generation
born. Now we expect to live to see how our offspring turn out
and more. In 1900 people in their forties had only a 10 percent
chance of having two living parents. In 1980, 40 percent of
Americans in their late fifties were still calling someone Mom
or Dad. And many of us will live to witness the sixty-fifth
birthdays of "our babies." In the 1980 census, 10 percent of
people over sixty-five had a child who was also over sixty-
five.[2]

Sociologists use the phrase "acceleration of the generational
wheels" to describe this change, the chance to know distant
generations and be adults together for decades that may be the
best gift our new longevity confers. But doing this also means
being a pioneer. New roles must be acted out: how to behave
as a mother to a "senior citizen" daughter; how to be
Grandma to a middle-aged corporation head.

In negotiating these uncharted generational waters, we can
get guidance from what others are doing. Are these new relationships working out? How are today's aging parents and
adult children getting along?

Children and Parents as Adults

One gerontological truth flies in the face of a widespread belief—that children and their aging parents must be less close
today than they used to be. Not so! In many ways the generations seem just as entwined now as they ever were.

In a set of studies done in 1957, 1963, and 1975, Ethel
Shanas, now professor emeritus of sociology at the University
of Illinois, compared how many times per week or month a
large national sample of adult children and their elderly parents visited or called one another.[3] Although we would expect
the amount of contact to have markedly declined over this period, stretching from the Eisenhower fifties to the liberated
seventies, there was little change. Children still lived close to
their parents, over three-fourths within a half-hour drive.
More than half had seen each other either that day or the day
before. About four in five had visited within the past week.
These statistics continue to apply in the late 1980s. Far from
being a nation of isolated nuclear families, intense contact between adult children and their elderly parents is typical of
American family life.

If parents live far away, they sometimes move closer to a
child when they develop physical problems. As I will describe
in more depth in the chapter on changing residence, this has
become a measurable demographic trend. People who left
their home states for a retirement home years earlier move
back to be near their children when frailty strikes.[4] Children,
anxious about worrying from a distance about an ailing
mother or father, often encourage the move. Or the push to be
close may be a more positive one.

*After my husband retired, we moved to Florida to be near my
eighty-year-old mother. We were lured by the sunshine and by
our fears for her health, and I missed her. I wanted to spend
these last precious years close by. At first we had a trying
time. I told her I'd go crazy if she kept calling to check in ten
times a day! We were adult enough to work things out. Now,
as mature ladies over sixty, we have the best of all mother/
daughter relationships: we are close friends.*

Over the past twenty years, as study after study has shown it to be false, gerontologists have tried to dispel what they call "the myth of family uninvolvement." To their bewilderment, the idea that Americans are neglecting their elderly parents survives intact. (Because it will not die, Shanas has called it a Hydra-headed monster.) Why does this idea seem so right?

One reason is probably that nursing homes have become such obvious features on the American landscape. What else could the boom in nursing-home care mean but people shirking their duty to sick parents, washing their hands of an obligation willingly assumed by children in every generation past?

But the estimated 1.5 million older Americans now living in nursing homes mask a less visible fact. At least twice as many severely disabled older people do not live in institutions as live in nursing homes. These people are usually being cared for by their families, often at great personal cost. Studies show that nursing-home placement is something most families work strenuously to avoid. When a person has living sons or daughters, it frequently happens as a last resort, when the older person's caretaker—frequently a daughter, sometimes elderly—becomes incapacitated herself.[5]

Nursing homes are really a testament not to filial neglect, but to the historic increase in the number of the very old—people who need a level of care unparalleled in the past. Today aged parents may need help for years with dressing, bathing, or getting around. For this generation of children, honoring the obligation to physically (and financially) care for parents in their declining years can be an overwhelming task.

According to Elaine Brody, an expert on family care, we tend to miss the fact that conditions are so different.[6] Equating then to now, children who have disabled elderly parents often feel chronically guilty about not doing everything; they feel like moral failures when they have to send their mothers or fathers to a nursing home. But, nursing-home placement may be a rational choice based on love, not an abandonment. Sometimes a nursing home can offer far better care than the most devoted attention any family could provide on its own.

Caregiving children also reproach themselves for not giving everything with a free heart, not realizing that caring for elderly parents has always been a job done as much out of obligation as from pure love.

In a thought-provoking 1985 article, psychologist William Jarrett argued that the idea that caring for aged parents should be a labor of love is a modern one.[7] Caring for parents in their old age always evoked mixed feelings, but like many things in life, it was a duty people shouldered without wondering over much about how they felt. However, in this era of liberation we have been conditioned to look askance at duty. ("We are not being true to ourselves if we do things we do not really want to do.") So we tell ourselves we should feel affectionate and rarely be resentful about the obligation of parent care. This pressure to feel in an emotionally "correct" way compounds the strain that today's caregiving children face. They torture themselves about not loving as much as they should, because in confusing duty with desire, they hold themselves to an emotional standard past generations never had to meet.

The idea that we care less is reinforced by another change in externals. Today parents and adult children are less likely to live in the same house than they were even a generation ago. In Shanas's 1957 survey, more than a third of the parents lived with their children. By 1975 the number had dropped dramatically, to only 18 percent.

However, it is the parents—more than the children—who want it that way. In the past, extended families lived together in large part because they could not afford to live separately.[8] Today, mainly because the older generation is better off financially, there is less economic necessity. Older people are usually averse to the idea of moving in with a child.[9]

My daughter wants me to sell my house and move in with her. I am smart enough to say no. I remember the fights and bad feelings during the years my mother lived with me. Our time as adults under one roof gave real meaning to the cliché "there can only be one boss." I want my independence, and I want to keep the good relationship we have. Although the depression forced my parents to move in with my husband and me, the problems with this arrangement are older than King Lear. No matter how much you trust your children, never give your life over to them.

A 1984 Canadian study shows that our ethnic background affects our willingness to share a household with our children. When researchers used census data to compare the living arrangements of older widowed women of Italian and Jewish descent, they found that, even controlling for income and number of offspring, the Italian women were much more likely to be living with a child than the Jewish widows.[10]

Although cultural background does make some difference, all things being equal, most people would probably still vote no to moving in. Our home is our castle, the place where we rule as independent adults. Who would freely relinquish his own rule to be—as is usually true of the older generation—a guest under someone else's roof? Also, living with a child smacks too much of being a burden. Many older people even prefer going to a nursing home to "intruding" on a daughter or son. But is it true that parents and children who live together pay an emotional price?

A study of Chicago families done about a decade ago by researchers at the University of Chicago implies they may.[11] The psychologists interviewed three generations separately— a young adult grandchild, a middle-aged father and mother, and one aged grandparent. They found that the small number of families who shared households were indeed emotionally worse off. Young married daughters living with middle-aged mothers in particular were rated more unhappy and immature. Although we do not know which is the chicken and which the egg—the families who lived together may have chosen to do so because they were already having more trouble handling life—this research shows that the risk of emotional problems may indeed be higher if the generations live under one roof.

Living together compounds the difficult transformation parents and their adult children must make—beginning with a lopsided relationship, ending with one that must be relatively equal to work well. We begin as dependent baby and all-powerful adult. We must completely change how we feel and act to get along as two equally competent human beings. We do have twenty years to accomplish this transformation. But we must fight inertia, the human tendency for patterns of relating to stay the same. So we often stay stuck as child and parent, fighting to be seen as different, carrying around feelings we had about each other from year one.

Family conflict is also more likely because parents and children are now encouraged to be "honest" with one another. Honest or open comments often are a code word for criticizing, saying something the other person should know but won't like. Although sometimes the older generation bears the brunt of a child's honesty, the impulse to correct usually flows the other way, causing the ageless complaint of grown-up children: "My parents treat me like a baby. They don't understand I'm an adult."

I am a doctor. I have a husband and children. When I visit my parents it takes only a day before I am reduced to a tearful little girl. The comments are relentless: "Haven't you gained a little weight? Let me take you shopping; I notice you don't have a really nice dress. Are you sure you should be working, not staying home with your son?" When I get angry, my mother doesn't understand: "You always took offense so easily as a child."

The study of the Chicago families lends scientific weight to this common complaint. Children resent their parents' advice giving because, no matter how old a child is, it continues to be the older generation who gives most of the advice.

The University of Chicago researchers wanted to explore what the different generations talked about. They used this technique: A set of cards was shown to each person, who was asked, "Do you and _____ talk about this?" If the answer was yes, the interviewer then asked whether the person had given or gotten advice about the subject from the other family member. The researchers were trying to discover what issues are "hot" topics for families. In what direction does advice flow between the generations?

Though advice flowed in both directions, the most frequent pattern remained the same. Whether a child was twenty or fifty-five, in relation to a parent he usually got more advice than he gave. The exception was when the parent generation was widowed or in bad health. Then advice giving became more equal or was reversed, the role of adviser shifting to the child. In other words, parents stand firm as parents no matter how old either they or their children are. It is only when a parent seems less capable—because of poor health or having to handle life without a spouse—that the much-feared role reversal seems to take place and the child takes over the adviser role.

In this study the "hot" topics for family advising tended to differ along sex-role lines. Fathers and grandfathers gave advice about work, education, and money. Mothers and grandmothers concentrated more on traditional "woman's" concerns—dating, how to get along with people, the importance of family and friends. When the men were asked why they did not attempt to advise about relationships, the oldest grandfather generation, who most often steered clear of these topics, seemed surprised: "Everyone knows these women's issues are none of men's business!"

And so, as we might imagine, the most delicate subjects for family discussion differed for men and women. For grandfathers and fathers the most sensitive topics were those in their advising domain: politics, race relations, social policy, work, money. For the women, "relationships" was the most touchy area. It was here that advising flowed fast and furious among mothers and daughters and grandmothers, and so here disagreements were most likely to flare up. Because of this, to keep harmony, the families reported that they sometimes had to develop conversational demilitarized zones and not talk too much about their concerns in these emotion-laden areas of life. Paradoxically, keeping close depended on keeping emotionally separate too.

Advising is perilous. The more of it we do, the greater the chance of having a fight. The very areas where we try to mold one another by being honest or instructing are those where we tend to have trouble getting along. At the same time, advising is also central to family life. Not only is it essential to raising children, advising is what gives families a coherent world vision, a shared life view. And even though the Chicago families fought, they were close, glued together by the common values that years of teaching one another can impart. But, to preserve their good feelings about one another, the adult generations had to learn a lesson: try to steer clear of touchy subjects; more often than you would like, hold your tongue.

ADVISING YOUR ADULT CHILD

Parents stay parents (teachers) for the best reasons. It is hard to keep quiet when speaking up might save your child from suffering—to watch from the sidelines when your son or daughter is doing something that seems certain to cause pain for years to come.

But the saying "people must make their own mistakes" is true. Giving your opinion on what an adult should do usually does not work unless the person is already 90 percent in agreement anyway. And even when children agree wholeheartedly, advice may make them angry because they are already trying desperately to do just what you suggest: "You should get married" (There's nothing I want more, but I'm ashamed to tell her that); "You should lose ten pounds" (I've tried every diet, but I'll be damned if I'll let him know); "You should get a better job" (I look through the want ads every day, but I'll never tell her I keep getting rejected in interviews). Unfortunately, these eminently reasonable suggestions are also intensely unhelpful. They rub salt in an open wound.

Having a good relationship with your children as adults means making an effort to act less like a parent and more like a friend. People who have mastered the art of friendship know to praise lavishly, be supportive and encouraging, and stifle many criticisms they are tempted to make. And good friends are like family—there in a crisis to help out. So when the impulse strikes to tell your children something for their own good, think carefully. Would you really be this frank if they were not your flesh and blood?

Since parenthood is different from friendship, on matters that vitally affect your child you will not want to keep silent. But you can try to get your message across in the best possible way. Rather than blindly criticizing ("You need to lose ten pounds"; "When are you getting married?"), offer something positive along with the pill, a concrete way of helping the per-

son change. Send a best-selling diet book or call with information about the local Weight Watchers group. Tell your daughter about that singles social at the church or ask Mrs. Jones if
her eligible son wants to meet a wonderful woman. Your child
may laugh ruefully at your "mothering" pressure but is more
likely to do what you suggest.

Avoid harping. If you are not being heard, raising the volume of your pleas will not help. It is more likely to get you
called a nag. If holding your tongue forever seems impossible,
resolve to keep quiet for a limited time: "I won't mention
Jane's weight when I see her next Tuesday." "This spring I'll
put a moratorium on those marriage questions." When you
have successfully kept mum until your limit, you might set
another limited silence vow. When the temptation to speak
gets strong, regain the proper perspective: "Would telling her
again really do any good?"

BEING ADULTS TOGETHER HAS BUILT-IN STRAINS

Sociologists Joseph Kuypers and Vern Bengston offer a deeper
analysis of why adult child/aging parent relationships can be
so troublesome.[12] There are three unspoken rules about family
life that parents and children tend to violate periodically as
they live together for decades as adults.

*Rule 1: As children grow up they need less parental attention
and care.* New parents are happy to be on call twenty-four
hours a day to an infant or a toddler, in part because they know
the overwhelming demands will gradually lessen. Children
grow up. The amount that must be given wanes over the
years. When children become adults, they leave and parents
can remake their own lives.

But though the normal order is toward less and less involvement, adult children sometimes want parents to give more in
times of need. Side by side with the expectation that parental
giving will wane is the idea that parents should always put
their children first. So children often feel hurt when they ask
for help and sense that their parents are unwilling. The older
generation feels different: "I no longer have to drop everything
at my child's whim. The time is over when his needs always
take precedence."

*I wanted to spend my Easter vacation in Florida with Mom and
Dad. When I called to make arrangements, my mother said an
old friend was visiting that week. We don't get to see one another that often. It would be hard to come at another time, and
shouldn't a son always come first over a friend? I'm not being
childish or demanding as she seems to feel. Parents should always put their children first.*

Arguments about priorities are most likely to flare up over
nonessential requests: "Will you baby-sit on Friday?" "Can I
use your pool next week?" In a crisis, when a child genuinely
must have help, the issue is clearer. Most parents want to step
in and give everything. The problem is when to step out. How
long should parents give "excessively"?

For instance, suppose your son leaves for college, graduates,
and then moves back in temporarily until he can find a job.
The temporary arrangement becomes permanent. The weeks
slide into months. You feel put upon but guilty. True, he is
making some money now, but not really enough to live well.
Yes, I want to be alone with my husband, but I would feel terrible kicking my own child out. Then imagine the guilt if your
child is also in real emotional pain—for instance, after a divorce.

Colleen Johnson of the University of California interviewed
middle-class San Francisco area women whose children had
recently been divorced.[13] She found that the demands on these
women were heavy but that they rose to the occasion, serving
as baby-sitters to the grandchildren, welcoming a suddenly
single son back home. Still, many were resentful at being saddled with unexpected parental obligations at this time of life.

*After my daughter was divorced she moved in with the chil-
dren, who are now eight and five. My husband has a heart condition. The children get on his nerves. We are upset at having
a family to care for in our old age. Joanne feels different. She
says it's my job to take her in for as long as it takes her to get
on her feet. I don't know how to reconcile the conflict; either I
suffer under a burden that has no end, or I feel terrible for not
reaching out to a child in need.*

What are some answers to this dilemma? Let's hold off on solutions until after describing the next two family rules. They also involve negotiating how responsible parents and children should be for one another as adults.

Rule 2: *When children marry, their loyalty shifts from the family they were born into to the family they create.* Rationally, elderly parents understand that their children have to put their own spouses and children "over" them. Because of the difficult asymmetry basic to being a parent, the heart can lag behind: our children stay first to us forever, but we ultimately must rank second in their lives.

"She's not repaying me for all the years I gave her" is the timeworn complaint that grows out of this inequity. Though some children do neglect their parents, the idea that reparations are necessary implies a parent has lost sight of what being a mother (or father) is all about. The essence of parenthood *is* giving more than you get. The truth is that your children are more important to you than you are to them. Accepting this natural imbalance in our importance is fairly easy when our life is full and happy, but when illness or isolation makes people needy, the yearning for equality may become intense. When a mother or father expects an equal commitment that should not be there, the most doting child weighs out deficient; resentment poisons the purest filial love.

My love for Mom is turning into frustration and guilt. No matter how much I show her I care, she accuses me of not giving enough. It came to a head when I took her out to dinner and then called the next day. Instead of "thanks for a lovely time," I heard, "Why is it you never come around?" I love her, but I cannot give her what she really wants—to be everything in my life.

The bottomless pit of this mother's need partly explains a puzzling research finding. Older people who see their adult children very often are no happier than those who see them less frequently.[14] What is important is not the quantity—how much time, or how many visits or calls—but the fit between what is expected and received. When we expect absolute devotion, even if we are getting almost everything we feel deprived.

A feeling of deprivation also comes about from mistakenly equating the past to now. If you remember your elderly mother's living with you, you may resent not living with your daughter, forgetting the reason you took Mom in: neither of you had the money to live separately. If you cared for your ill mother on your own, you may be angry that your daughter has hired an attendant, not realizing your mother never needed as much help bathing and dressing as you do. The same applies to another dramatic cultural change. As of 1980, only 1 percent of Americans were giving their parents heavy financial support, very unlike the situation in any past generation.[15]

In a 1985 article Daniel Callahan, director of the Hastings Center for the Study of Ethical Issues, spelled out the obvious reason.[16] There is less need. The government, not our children, now provides for us financially in our old age. He quotes an insightful person who extols the virtues of that arrangement in this way:

> We (older folks) don't like to take money from our kids. We don't want to be a burden. They don't like giving us money either. We all get angry at each other if we do it that way. So, we all sign a political contract to deal with what anthropologists would call the intergenerational transfer of wealth. The young people give money to the government. I get money from the government. That way we can both get mad at the government and keep on loving one another.[17]

Federal spending on the elderly, which has nearly doubled since 1960, is succeeding in freeing this generation of older people from depending on their children's charity. In fact, in 1984 older people were less likely to have incomes below the poverty level than the nation as a whole (if we include children). While the national poverty rate was 14.7 percent that year, for people over sixty-five it was only 12.4 percent.[18]

Not only has Uncle Sam helped boost the elderly out of poverty, Callahan agrees that this government takeover does further family harmony. Children should not be put in the difficult position of choosing whether to give to their children or their parents, or of giving to their parents at the price of impoverishing themselves in their own old age.

But even though most parents probably rejoice at not having to take a nickel from their children, the difference from the past can hurt. An aged father remembers the check he dutifully delivered to his parents, chafing because his forty-year-old son is not offering or even accepting money. However, his son is just following Kuypers and Bengston's third family rule. **Rule 3:** *Parents give to their children and not the reverse.* Having to violate this rule causes a family universal pain. What child wants to see his mother or father diminished? What parent wants to feel the humiliation of depending on a child? We also have compelling evidence that the nursing job is more stressful when it is done by a child rather than by a husband or wife. When University of California researchers compared spouse and child caregivers, they found that though husbands and wives were distressed about what was happening, they usually did not feel resentful. In fact, many said their marriages had gotten closer as they were thrust into this difficult situation. But if the caregiver was a child, the reaction was often quite different. The older person's demands caused conflict, the relationship deteriorated, competing demands from the caregiver's family added to the pressure, and children emotionally distanced themselves—either by going into therapy or by deciding "I can't stand it anymore" and turning completely to paid help.[19]

What does the person on the receiving end feel when this change occurs in the natural order of giving? To answer this question, Lucy Rose Fisher of the University of Minnesota compared the feelings of a small group of physically disabled older parents and their caretaking children.[20] The two were upset about different things. The children were quick to label what was happening a "role reversal." Parents did not mention, or give any sign they were troubled by, the change in roles. They were deeply distressed about being physically dependent, no longer able to "go out on my own." Their children mourned the mental loss they saw.

It sounds terrible to say, I guess, but I could have handled the fact that Dad was in pain, because you can control pain with medication, better than the fact that he wasn't himself. He wasn't the person I remembered him as being—the caring, lovable person he once was. That was harder for me to deal with than knowing he had cancer and was probably going to die soon.

In this study the main emotion the children had was grief, not resentment or annoyance about shouldering what was often a twenty-four-hour job. So the feelings of caregiving children actually vary greatly. Although caring for an ill parent is almost always upsetting, children differ dramatically in how put-upon they feel. Surprisingly, when the burden seems intolerable, the job itself tends not to be the main cause.

Kuypers and Bengston suggest that children are most likely to feel overwhelmed and resentful when they look to the future and see no end in sight. It is the thought of forever that tends to transform caring for a parent from a labor of love (or a duty willingly accepted) into a crushing burden.

In studying families coping with dementia, psychologist Steve Zarit of Penn State University finds that caregivers tend to feel most stressed when they are simultaneously squeezed by other *unexpected* demands: a sick husband, an adult child still in the house. And his research shows that people feel most overwhelmed when they feel their family and friends are unsupportive.[21] If everyone else says "put Mom in a nursing home," or if brothers and sisters seem to be shirking their responsibility, then parent care seems exhausting and unbearable. In other words, a burden that falls unfairly feels heaviest.

The job itself is not irrelevant. Does your mother have Alzheimer's disease? Is she physically or verbally abusive, incontinent, prone to wake up and wander during the night? Caregiving children find coping with this illness and its difficult symptoms particularly hard. And the past looms large. A lifelong loving parent/child relationship seems to provide a reserve of good feeling that greatly lightens the stress.[22]

THE IMPLICATIONS FOR GETTING ALONG

If you and a parent or child are embroiled in conflict, think about your trouble on a more academic plane. Is your problem due to clashing expectations or violations of any of these family rules? Pinpoint the source of your anger. Consider the situation from the other person's perspective. Understand that having contrasting feelings is normal to being adult pioneers together.

Perhaps you can use this chapter as a way of clearing the air. Ask your child or parent to read the sections that relate directly to your problem and to think about things from your point of view. Use the scientific distance offered by my rational analysis to help keep your "meeting of the minds" from becoming a shouting match.

Approach differences with the idea that you are both right. Neither of you is giving too little or asking too much. It is the contradictions inherent in being adults together that are to blame. Work out a compromise between your needs with this idea in mind. Preserving your love is more important than "winning" any argument.

Remember, discomfort, anger, and resentment are common when the normal rules of giving and getting are breached and one person needs "too much." What can you do if you are in this difficult situation? For instance, suppose your parent or child needs an unusual degree of help and you want to give, but in the most emotionally comfortable way?

Before you get involved, decide exactly what you can and cannot do. Write down the things you can comfortably do and those jobs that would be too much, including the time you can commit to helping plus the specific tasks you can manage well: "I would be able to visit Jane three times a week; I could shop and baby-sit while she looks for a job." Then, in another column, list the requests you cannot fulfill: "I would feel resentful if I had to watch the children every day; it would be a real deprivation to lend her my car." Do the most you can, but be clear about your limits. Resentfully doing more is likely to cause both you and the other person grief.

Try not to feel guilty about your limit, even if outsiders say your commitment is wrong. We all have different set points, different valid priorities in life.

Whereas we think the world will judge us only for doing too little, people surprisingly often are criticized for doing too much. For instance, children are frequently pressured by doctors, friends, and other relatives to send their parents to a nursing home, accused of being martyrs if they resist. But the actions others see as martyrdom may be emotionally just right for them. They would feel more uncomfortable *not* taking care of their flesh and blood themselves.

Kuypers and Bengston suggest that resentment is most likely when a commitment seems open ended. So it may help you to give with a freer heart and define your limits better if you know how long the person will need your help. If your relative is ill, make an appointment to discuss the situation with the doctor. "How is the illness likely to progress? What kind of help is needed now? What will be needed later on?"

My mother has liver cancer and may live only a year. I have been flying down to New York from my home in Boston to visit her every weekend. Since I work and have young children, I am exhausting myself, even though I want to be with her as much as I can. I thought I would give her every Saturday and Sunday. I'm changing my mind. I'll go slower now and save my strength for the time she really needs me, so I can give her everything then.

If your relative is likely to need more and more as the months pass, pace your involvement now so you can be there when you are needed most. If the time frame of your help is undefined (Do you fly in to help your daughter with the new baby for a week or a month? How long can your daughter stay with you after her divorce?), set your own limit: "I can take a week off from work to help." "She and the children can stay for a month." Mentally define your limit before you board the plane or before she and the children move in.

Communicate your plan clearly. Then diplomatically tell both your relative and other family members exactly what you have decided: "I will help with A, B, and C, but I cannot do X, Y, and Z"; "I can baby-sit every Saturday and in emergencies, but not every time you go out"; "I'm thrilled to have you stay here, but I expect you to find your own place by April 1." Having a clear shared understanding and a structured commitment minimizes the resentment predictable with an open-ended arrangement. If whether and when you visit is up in the air, Mom will wonder every day if you are coming. She will be upset when she makes her morning call and you "reject" her by saying you have other plans. You, in turn, will feel continually pressured—guilty when you say "not today," put upon by an obligation that has to seem excessive just because it is always there.

If your limit is less than the person wants, explain why it is impossible for you to do more. If you are sharing the helping with several other family members, explain the reasons for your limit to each of them individually. Rather than leaving people in the dark and risking being labeled ungiving, let everyone know why your other obligations make it impossible to do more.

If the price of sticking to your set point is just ill feeling, be open to change. If your ninety-four-year-old mother would like you to visit twice a week, reconsider your once-a-week maximum if she is deeply upset about your not being there the extra day. Maybe a compromise would work. You might come two mornings a week rather than one full day. If your sister accuses you of dumping your responsibility for Dad on her because you live far away and she lives close by, stifle your impulse to slam down the phone. Be sisterly. You cannot be on the spot to help, but perhaps every few months you could bring Dad for extended vacations at your house. Negotiate, keeping your eye on what is important. Sometimes it is better to do more than we want in order to preserve our family's love and our good feelings about ourselves for years to come.

Be alert to the effect of your help: Are you genuinely doing good? A hidden danger in being a giver is doing too much. Taking over looks so right, but it may do more harm than good. For instance, your mother is having trouble walking to the store, so you do her weekly shopping. Soon she gets more and more depressed. Though shopping was a physical strain, for her mental health she needed that push to get out of the house.

Giving too much is seductive because it can be so satisfying. Both people may feel wonderful about their arrangement even though it is wrong. For example, you adore having your daughter and grandchildren around and she loves being there, but living with you is bad for her. It is keeping her from making a new life after her divorce. To really be helpful you should be encouraging her to move out, even at the price of risking her anger and depriving yourself.

People of any age are vulnerable to developing excess disabilities, the disease of incapacity produced by being helped too much (see chap. 1). Before rushing in to take over, remember that loving is not the same as giving everything; sometimes the best love lies in giving less. To determine if you are being genuinely helpful, ask yourself these questions: "Is my daughter more independent now than before I started helping her out?" "In what specific ways is what I am doing enriching Dad's life?" "What are my goals in helping? Are they being reached?" In other words, to know whether you are doing the right thing, look at the results.

Another pitfall in giving is depriving someone of the best care by feeling it is your responsibility to do everything yourself: refusing to hire an attendant because caring for a mother is a daughter's obligation; nursing a sick daughter devotedly rather than hiring the trained nurse she needs. Be careful to gear your helping not to your morality ("family is best"), but to your loved one's needs.

Your job is to short-circuit the downward spiral I described earlier. A child starts out doing everything, becomes more and more resentful and unhappy, and finally gives up totally in frustration and rage. If you see this pattern taking shape, act to stop it before it reaches its predictable end—hating your parent (or child) and hating yourself.

Now suppose you are on the receiving end. How can you ask for more in the best possible way? How can you tell if you are asking too much?

Clarify what you need and assess how reasonable your requests are. If necessary, list your needs and rank them according to priority. "What help is critical, and what things can I do on my own? Can some of these jobs be done by people other than my daughter or son?" Put a check after the essentials and resolve to ask your family for help only with them.

If you feel your children are being ungiving, think carefully. "Is it really complete devotion I want? Is it possible, given their other commitments, for my family to do all these things for me?" Do not expect the impossible. Although you are upset by your daughter's making her husband and children her first priority, it is right for you to rank second. Would you really feel good about your job as a parent if you raised a child who put *your* needs first?

Communicate what you need clearly. Carefully spell out

what you want. Do not say nothing and then be upset because your family has not guessed your needs. If you want more attention, you extend the invitations. Invite your daughter over; don't wait passively for her call. If you need help with shopping, *tell* your son. You cannot blame people for being ungiving unless they know what to give.

If you ask for something and are refused, keep a sense of proportion. When your family can't visit, it need not mean they don't care; it may just be impossible to get away now. Do you know the pressures they are under, what is happening in the rest of their lives? It is human nature to be oversensitive when we are on the receiving end. Do not let your feelings of vulnerability make you read total rejection into what is really a minor "not right now."

Be wary of taking behavior reflecting cultural change as a personal affront. When you fume, "I took Mom in, and Sara should do the same for me," look around. "What are Mrs. X's children doing? Is living together really a good benchmark of daughterly devotion? Am I using an outmoded standard to assess her love?"

A study of 753 older people shows how demoralizing being on the receiving end can be.[23] Eleanor Stoller of the State University of New York found that the people she studied who got help from their families tried to reciprocate in some way. When they could not balance the getting with at least some giving, they tended to be depressed.

So if you have to accept help, try to give something in return. If you cannot leave your house, could you help your daughter do some of her chores by phone? Could you bake, knit, help financially? Ask your child to come up with ways you can be helpful. If she says "I don't need anything," persist. Explain that you need to reciprocate for your own self-esteem.

If your family is neglecting you, avoid browbeating them. Cajoling, recriminations, and guilt-inducing strategies will make things worse. If possible, put a temporary cast on what is happening: "They have not failed me; they just cannot give me what I need right now." Look for more hospitable baskets to put your emotional eggs in. Focus on your friends or on other relatives. Turning to other people for comfort and help will not stop the hurt, but it should lessen it.

Grandparents

Being a grandparent is different from practically every other relationship we have in life. Normally we are loved for our achievements, the content of what we do. Grandparents are important in a way that overshadows the calls, the visits, or the presents. They are loved for a more elusive quality—just being Grandma or Grandpa.

My three-year-old son sees my mother only every six months. He hardly speaks to her at all. But when he feels bad (or angry at us), he calls wildly for her. Her distant involvement doesn't matter. She is everything to him just because she is his grandma—not anything else.

Gerontologist Lillian Troll calls grandparents "the family watchdogs."[24] Even though they normally stand in the wings, they are poised to step forward in a crisis. Grandchildren sense their crucial value early on. They are the family safety net. A good example is when a daughter with children is going through a divorce. In this crisis even distant grandparents often become heavily involved; they visit, comfort, take the grandchildren more often. Their shrouded importance is illuminated, their hidden value clear.

Grandparents also help their grandchildren by helping their daughters and sons. In reviewing the research, Gunhild Hagestad of Northwestern University cites a study showing that if a young mother was close to her mother, she felt more at ease and more competent being a mother herself.[25] In other words, grandparents help their grandchildren by helping their children become better parents.

My daughter Sara, who lives in Michigan, is giving birth in September and I'm flying there to help. Though I've forgotten almost everything about new babies myself, we'll both be there to muddle through. I hope my presence will make her less anxious and get her off to a good start. Even though I'm nervous about being called in as "the expert," I can't wait!

Grandparents also can be family mediators, helping parents and children resolve their differences. Hagestad describes a study showing that adolescent girls often took their troubles with Mom to Grandma. These grandmothers had unique leverage. Not only were they a shoulder to cry on, but they helped smooth over the conflict by gently interpreting the parent's point of view to the child.

Grandparents are the family cement; the glue that keeps the extended family close; the reason sisters and brothers come to see one another on holidays or at special times. This crucial cementing function may become obvious only when a grandparent dies.

When my mother passed away, I lost my sister and her family as well. Christmas had been a tradition in our house since I was a little girl. Everyone trekked to my parents' house for their annual party even though going meant putting off our vacation plans for a few days. This Christmas, the first since my mother's death, I decided to carry on the tradition and have the party myself. But without Mom, my sister decided she didn't have to come and booked plane reservations to Florida instead.

Here is Hagestad's summary of the ways grandparents enrich a grandchild's life:

Grandparents serve—as symbols of connectedness within and
    between lives;
as people who can listen and have the time to do so;
as reserves of time, help, and attention;
as links to the unknown past;
as people who are sufficiently varied, flexible, and complex to
    defy
easy categories and clear-cut roles.

Understanding that what grandparents symbolize is as important as what they do, let's look at Hagestad's last statement. What are the varied, flexible, and complex styles of being a grandparent?

STYLES OF GRANDPARENTING

Grandparents share a clear idea of what they are supposed to be like, if only to distinguish it from how they really behave.

When University of California sociologist Colleen Johnson asked middle-class, middle-aged grandmothers to describe the grandmother stereotype, she got the same answer: a frail lady who knits booties by the hearth. Most women rejected this Currier and Ives portrait as having nothing to do with them. Many said they felt more like a "pal" to their grandchildren. Sharing experiences was important. Visits to McDonald's or even the disco supplanted grandmotherly goodies from the oven.[26]

Today the grandmother stereotype is genuinely outmoded—more likely to fit great- or even great-great-grandmothers. In an age when most people become grandparents in their vigorous early fifties, the elderly lady by the fire has been replaced by a figure much less wooden and removed—a person who has the energy and motivation to be centrally involved with her grandchildren for decades in an unprecedented way.

Actually, far from every grandparent is close and involved. People choose to interpret one of life's most undefined roles in a variety of ways. In a classic quarter-century-old study, researchers found these distinct grandparenting styles.[27]

The formal grandparent. This person saw the grandchildren regularly, but at defined times such as the first Sunday of each month. The relationship was formal, one of grandparent and grandchild, not friends. Activities were traditional—bringing presents, going to the circus.

The surrogate parent. This person was extremely involved, sharing child rearing with the parent. Surrogate parents babysat daily or visited for hours at least several times a week. Often they lived in a grandchild's house.

The distant figure. This type of grandparent was the opposite of the surrogate parent—very uninvolved, seeing the grandchildren briefly and infrequently.

A person's age affected grandparenting style. Older grandparents, those over sixty-five, were most likely to be formal grandparents or distant figures. Younger grandparents were more likely to be "pals" or heavily involved.

More recent research agrees that age is one factor that determines a person's grandparenting style. When sociologists Andrew Cherlin and Frank Furstenberg studied 510 grandparents with teenage grandchildren, they found that younger grandparents were indeed more likely to be very involved.[28]

Older grandparents tended to be more removed, probably because younger grandparents are more apt to be "younger in thinking" and also in better health. They have the energy to be close.

About half of this national sample of grandparents was very involved—seeing a grandchild frequently, sometimes serving as a confidant. This is particularly encouraging because these were grandparents of adolescents; and just as parenthood follows the principle of waning involvement, grandparenthood often does too.

I was so disappointed in the last visit I had with my grandson. I wanted to stay and talk, but he was just interested in getting out to a baseball game. I remember how his eyes used to light up when he was two and I would arrive. I know the older he gets the more he has to have his own life—It's almost like I'm going through the empty nest again.

However, Cherlin and Furstenberg also found that the categories "close" or "uninvolved" grandparent don't universally apply. A grandparent's closeness often differed tremendously from grandchild to grandchild. Grandparents have favorites, the grandchildren they feel temperamentally closest to. Closeness also depends on physical proximity. It is natural to be more involved with a grandchild living around the block than one a six-hour plane ride away. And no matter how involved grandparents want to be, their closeness depends on another factor—the wishes of the generation in between.

THE FRUSTRATIONS OF BEING A GRANDPARENT

Being a grandparent is frustrating because you love but lack control. This lack of control is exemplified by "the norm of noninterference" that American grandparents usually say they try to abide by: "Do not meddle in how the grandchildren are being raised."[29] People may arrive at this golden rule of grandparenting out of experience, knowing the price of overstepping its bounds.

After my last visit to my parents in Rhode Island, I said "never again." My mother continually told me I wasn't being strict

*enough. She criticized the children's table manners and the
way they were dressed. She even expected my toddler to sit
quietly and play alone. The last day she knew there was trouble and tried to make amends. For the first time she told me
how cute the children were. I think she knows. It will be a
long time before we ever go back.*

Grandparents are vulnerable. Their access to their grandchildren depends on the goodwill of the parent generation. So
bad feelings with a son or daughter, a divorce, or even a child's
decision to move the family across the country can deprive
them of the contact they want. Parents of sons are most at
risk, because the mother usually determines a family's social
life. Because she naturally prefers her own parents, being a paternal grandparent often means being in second place.

The education in being second starts at the beginning, when
a daughter-in-law asks her mother, not her husband's mother,
for help in the weeks after a first grandchild's birth. It can continue through many Thanksgiving dinners and hoped-for invitations to the children's house.

*On holidays my daughter-in-law gets together with her par-
ents, only sometimes inviting my husband and me. Before he
got married my son and I were close. Now he lets his wife
make the social plans. She wants to be with her own mother; I
am left out.*

American families have what sociologists call a matrifocal
tilt. The generations are usually more closely knit on the
mother's side. Sons tend to separate from their parents more
easily; daughters care more about staying close. Family ties
are usually stronger along maternal lines.[30] The way the matrifocal tilt of the family works against paternal grandparents
is sometimes heartbreakingly evident after a bitter divorce.
When the wife gets custody, a son's parents may be forbidden
to see their grandchildren again.

A fascinating 1987 study of middle-class mothers of divorced children shows that to keep the bond they have with
their grandchildren, mothers of sons seem to make a special
effort to preserve the relationship with their former daughters-
in-law. While 36 percent of the paternal grandmothers studied

saw a former daughter-in-law at least once a week, only 9 percent of the maternal grandmothers saw a former son-in-law. In other words, to preserve their access to the grandchildren, mothers of divorced sons may be unable to side just with their "own child" after a marriage breaks up. They have to remain friendly with the person who controls that access—the person who has custody, usually their former daughter-in-law.[31]

GETTING MORE SATISFACTION OUT OF BEING A GRANDPARENT

Being a grandparent is fraught with contradictions. You are close, and yet your hands are tied. Even "surrogate parents" who help bring up a grandchild come in at a child's invitation. They know there is only one true parent in the house. Grandparents follow the norm of noninterference because it works. *Criticizing grandchildren or their upbringing is more likely to provoke anger and distance than to bring constructive change.*

Being accepting (even when you feel like correcting) will help win the access to your grandchildren you want. When the impulse to make a negative comment strikes, think: "How will my daughter respond to what I am about to say? Would having a more disciplined grandchild be worth making her feel incompetent so she wants to run from me?"

Suppose you are careful to be very accepting yet still long for more contact than you are getting now. If you have not already done so, try these tactics: Ask your daughter or son if there are times you can help with the grandchildren. Be genuinely helpful when you visit, rather than having to be entertained. And instead of waiting to be invited to their house, ask the grandchildren to yours more often.

Be empathic when they do come. If they are toddlers, put away your precious crystal rather than continually yelling "Don't touch." Keep some toys around. Don't insist that young grandchildren sit through your lovingly cooked four-course meal. If your grandchildren are older, take them to interesting places such as the theater or a basketball game. Try to ensure that being with you is not an obligation, but a genuine treat.

Living far away presents special barriers. Could you set up

special times to fly there or have the grandchildren visit you? Might you encourage your son or daughter to take a family vacation at a resort halfway between your homes and meet them there? Would you feel comfortable coming to baby-sit while your daughter and son-in-law went on a second honeymoon? Use your creativity to see more of your grandchildren in a way that makes things easiest for everyone.

If your child is divorced and does not have custody of the children, the barrier to being close is even greater. You need to swallow any ill feelings and keep up a good relationship with your former son-in-law or (more likely) daughter-in-law. The message of the study just described is that success is possible. Many people are able to stay close. In fact, paternal grandparents in this touchy situation have one side benefit. The researchers who did this study found that though after a divorce the family network of maternal grandmothers tended to shrink because these women often broke contact with their former sons-in-law, for paternal grandmothers a child's divorce and remarriage often meant an enlargement of family ties. Why? Not only had these women kept up their relationships with their former daughters-in-law, they added another relative when their sons took new wives.

If you are a grandparent whose actual involvement seems frustratingly small, remember that as long as you love your grandchildren and are accepting and see them at least sometimes, you are likely to be valued more than you know. As ''family watchdog'' you symbolize what family is all about: a reliable, safe haven of last resort.

For More Information

ABOUT TAKING CARE OF AN AGED PARENT

Family Caregivers Program, National Council on the Aging, 600 Maryland Avenue S.W., West Wing 100, Washington, D.C. 20024. Central resource for families caring for disabled older relatives. Serves as a clearinghouse for information, publishes materials, advocates public policy offering support to caregivers.

Horne, J. *Caregiving: Helping an Aging Loved One.* Mount Prospect, Ill.: Scott, Foresman and AARP Books, 1985.

Guide for caregivers covering everything from handling legal affairs, to getting others involved, to handling the older person's emotional needs and your own. Also covers community services.

ABOUT GRANDPARENTHOOD

Bengston, V., and J. Robertson, eds. *Grandparenthood.* Beverly Hills, Calif.: Sage, 1985.
Though this is a book for professionals, it may be interesting to any intelligent reader. It offers a summary of current research and theory on grandparenthood.

Cherlin, A., and F. Furstenberg. *The New American Grandparent: A Place in the Family, a Life Apart.* New York: Basic Books, 1986.
The results of the first nationwide study of grandparents. Provides a detailed portrait of grandparenthood in America.

Kornhaber, A., and K. L. Woodward. *Grandparent/Grandchild: The Vital Connection.* Garden City, N.Y.: Anchor Books, 1981.
Describes interviews with grandparents illustrating the authors' thesis that the bond between grandparents and grandchildren is very important. Forcefully advocates the importance of being an involved grandparent.

TRANSITIONS

CHAPTER

6

RETIREMENT

For me the words "golden years" are not a sham. They fit the way I feel about this time of life. I built up my printing business from the beginning. I have my health and enough money to live. Though I was not forced to retire at sixty-five, the scramble for clients became too much. I didn't have the energy to go door to door. I never liked that exhibitionist partner of mine, though I tolerated him for thirty years. Getting old made his shenanigans unbearable; it was a relief to say goodbye. Still, I was afraid of being retired with cause. It has taken me more than a year and a half to find the life that's right. After a few months, the thrill of sleeping late wore off. I floundered, searching for things that would give purpose to my week. I tried tennis, swimming, volunteering at a hospital, and taking a course. I got depressed. Was there anything that could excite me? When I thought things through, I came up with a surprising answer: Do something similar to my old line of work. Use my carefully built-up skills, but without jumping headlong into the rat race. Do something low key, socially fulfilling, and very part time. Luckily, a friend suggested SCORE (Service Corps of Retired Executives).

As a SCORE volunteer I am using my talents, am helping others, and have latitude about how many hours I donate. I am a consultant three days a week to small companies that are struggling to get off the ground. I give advice about all aspects of management—marketing, advertising, training new staff. My opinions are respected. I am relaxed yet involved, kept energized to enjoy the other perks of this lovely age—to play tennis, swim, take a course—to do what I want when I want.

Along with this century's dramatic rise in life expectancy has come an increase in the years we devote to life's three major activities: education, work, and retirement. Children are spending more time in school; men and women in their middle years are spending more years working; and older people are spending much more time in retirement. The most striking change in how we spend our lives has been the evolution of retirement as our third life stage.[1]

At the turn of the century, life was made up of school and work. Men, having a life expectancy of 46.3 years, on average spent 1.2 years retired. Making up only 3 percent of the typical man's life, retirement was a brief interlude before death. By 1980 the average man spent almost 14 years as a retiree, a full 20 percent of his 69.3 years. Not only had retirement become a full-fledged stage of life, but a man could expect to spend more years in this third life stage than he did in the first.

Our retirement years have increased at the expense of our working years, not our school years. Whereas in 1980 the typical man spent five more years working than in 1900, the portion of his life spent in the labor force declined from 69 percent to 55 percent. (Because of their unprecedented entry into the job market during the 1970s, the figures are totally different for women. In 1900 American women worked outside the home an average of 6.3 years—about 13 percent of their life spans; in 1980 they could expect to spend more than a third of life working—27.5 years.)

Two influences have shaped the evolution of retirement as an American institution: the lure of being able to live without collecting a paycheck and the prod of mandatory retirement laws.

Although the Social Security Act passed in 1935 made leaving work at age sixty-five financially possible, retirement became fully palatable economically for many older workers only about twenty years ago. From 1968 to 1971 Congress raised Social Security benefits by 43 percent while prices increased by only 27 percent. In 1972 benefits were increased by another 20 percent. During the 1970s pension plans also proliferated (today they cover about one in three retirees).

These changes had a dramatic impact on the economic status of older people. From an alarming poverty rate of 28.5 per-

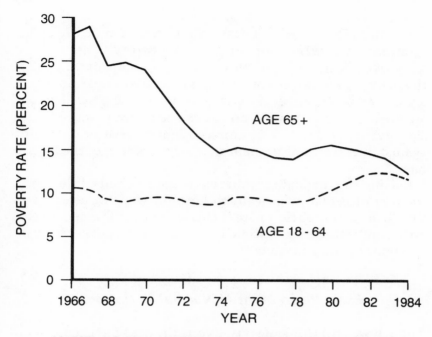

SOURCE: U.S. Bureau of the Census, Current Population Surveys, 1967-85.

Figure 3   Poverty rates for older versus younger adults, 1966–1984

cent in 1966, the number of people over sixty-five living below
the poverty line was more than halved by 1974, to 14.6 percent (compared with a poverty rate of 8.5 percent for adults
aged eighteen to sixty-four). Since then this decline has slowly
continued, while the proportion of younger adults living in
poverty has risen, causing the gap between old and young to
close (see fig. 3). In 1984, 12.4 percent of the elderly were living below the poverty line, while 11.7 percent of adults under
sixty-five and 14.7 percent of the nation as a whole (if we include children) were doing so.

Retirement has also become an American fact of life by
force. As small family businesses succeeded and grew into
large firms, employers needed to build in a way to let younger
workers advance and to gracefully get rid of older employees
who were too expensive or could no longer perform. Their solution was usually to institute mandatory retirement—fixed
company policies requiring all employees to retire by age
sixty-five.

But in 1978, when Congress passed the Amended Age Discrimination in Employment Act, mandatory retirement at sixty-five became illegal. Now, unless a company has fewer than twenty employees or a person is in an occupation where age can critically affect the work—or in certain cases if people are high-level executives—no one can be forced to retire before age seventy. (As of 1987, thirteen states have prohibitions against mandatory retirement that are stricter than the federal one.)

Raising the mandatory retirement age has helped the small fraction of people who want to keep on working after sixty-five. It has done little to stem the retirement stampede. Not only is retirement as entrenched a life stage as ever, so is retirement before sixty-five.

Early Retirement Is Normal Retirement

Though we still think of sixty-five as the age when people normally retire, the real retirement age has inched down. A 1978 Harris poll showed just how wide of the mark our traditional age, sixty-five, really is. Almost two-thirds of the national sample of retirees Harris polled had left work before age sixty-five; the true average American retirement age turned out to be only 60.6.[2]

Will the recent efforts to tinker with Social Security raise this age? Not really, according to a study conducted by the National Commission for Employment Policy. In 1983 major modifications in the Social Security Act were enacted to try to discourage retirement: gradually raising the age for collecting full benefits from sixty-five to sixty-seven by 2027; increasing the yearly bonus for people who retire late from 3 percent to 8 percent; reducing the fraction of benefits that retirees can get at age sixty-two from 80 percent to 70 percent by 2022. Unfortunately, the commission calculated that the net effect of these changes is likely to be surprisingly small, raising the average retirement age by only a few months.[3] Today health, the widespread availability of private and public pensions, expectations, and long-held plans are much more important in influencing the decision to retire than is Social Security. Although Social Security revved up the retirement engine, it is now fueled by other sources. What does power this critical decision of life?

The Decision to Retire

The most accurate information we have on why people decide to retire early (or late), and the effect of that decision on physical, financial, and emotional well-being, comes from a synthesis of the best retirement studies published by a team of gerontologists at Duke University in 1985.[4] From the hundreds of studies of retirement that have been done over the past quarter-century, the Duke social scientists selected seven to analyze. The studies they chose were comprehensive, exploring retirement in various ethnic and socioeconomic groups. They also were longitudinal, capturing the process of retirement over time. Instead of interviewing people at a single point either before or after leaving work, hundreds (or thousands) of workers nearing retirement age were picked and then questioned repeatedly over the next years.

The Retirement History Survey sponsored by the Social Security Administration is a good example of this ambitious type of research. In 1969 a representative nationwide sample of about twelve thousand male and unmarried female workers aged fifty-eight to sixty-three was selected and then reinterviewed every two years over the next decade (until 1979) as they gradually retired. Combining the results of this study with those of the others gives us answers to fascinating questions such as these: What motivates American workers to retire early or to go on working after age sixty-five? How does retiring affect people economically, psychologically, and physically?

EARLY RETIREMENT

In 1984, almost 90 percent of men and 60 percent of women in their early fifties were either working or looking for jobs. Among people turning sixty, the numbers were dramatically lower—68 percent and 40 percent. This trend toward leaving work as early as our late fifties has been gathering steam during the second half of this century, mirroring the historic expansion in Social Security and pensions. For instance, from 1950 to 1984 the percentage of men aged fifty-five to sixty-four in the labor force declined precipitously, from 88 percent to 64 percent.[5]

The main reason people give for leaving work early is financial. They retire because they can afford to live without collecting a paycheck. But why is taking the option to retire early so compelling? The reason is that over this past quarter-century our feelings about retiring have totally changed.

The New Lure of Retirement

When it comprised those few predeath years of infirmity, retirement was symbolic of the end of life. Able-bodied men collected paychecks. Retirement was the time when a person was put out to pasture because he could no longer perform. As people became able to retire in relative economic comfort, the emotional connotations attached to retirement changed. The pasture began to look greener and greener. From a tragedy, retirement was transformed into the time of life people were working *for*.

Today this new emotion is the winner. Surveys show that most American workers look forward to retirement. Even people who love their jobs vote yes to the idea of eventually not having to work.[6] But looking forward to retiring in the future is very different from giving up an activity that has filled our lives for all of adulthood. Why is it easy for so many people to take the step so early?

One reason may be that we begin preparing emotionally much earlier. In a 1985 study of 816 Boston-area men, the long-standing belief among retirement specialists—that people don't really plan for retirement—was stood on its head.[7] In contrast to previous studies that measured preparation by structured activities such as attending preretirement seminars, Linda Evans, David Ekerdt, and Raymond Bosse focused on more informal signs: How often did a man discuss retirement with his wife, relatives, or retired friends? How often did he read articles about retirement?

Although the intensity of thinking, reading, and discussing steadily increased as retirement time approached, even men who saw leaving work as a good fifteen years away did a good deal of planning for their retirement lives.

Fantasizing about retirement may help ease the anxiety attached to taking the plunge. The change from worker to retired person is much less wrenching if we have been there in spirit over the years. But a deeper explanation for why *men* are often so willing to leave even desirable, high-status jobs years before they have to may lie in personality—the emotional transformation that psychologists such as Carl Jung believe takes place after midlife.

According to these psychologists, once men reach middle age the success drive—the youthful lust for power—tends to erode. Maturity (and having tasted power) dims the excitement of moving and shaking. Retirement-oriented values take top priority—relaxing, enjoying relationships, focusing on family.[8]

Although not all psychologists agree that men do change in this way as they age, I saw firsthand evidence that older men view working differently at a seminar I attended on job seeking after retirement. Not one of the men in the audience raised his hand when the group leader asked if "status or power" would be an important consideration in their choosing to take a certain job. These elderly job seekers desperately wanted to work, but for the pleasure and the money, not for the sense of power a job might provide. Had I been in a room full of thirty-year-olds, the vote probably would have gone very much the other way.

A study done in the late 1960s in a small California town[9] suggested that having a more relaxed, relationship-oriented approach may make the late fifties and early sixties an especially happy time of life for men. Researchers at the University of California interviewed residents of the town at four pivotal ages—late adolescence, the early thirties, the mid-forties and the early sixties, at the brink of retirement. They found that the oldest men, interested in enjoying their families, not struggling to establish themselves or grasp for personal success, were happier than almost any other group.

However, the work ethic dies hard; the terror of just relaxing persists. So, as retirement specialist David Ekerdt suggested in a provocative 1986 article, to get ourselves to retire without guilt we have had to evolve a new national retirement ethic that stresses "busyness."[10] By "keeping as busy and involved as ever," retirees prove they have not been put out to pasture and are not "over the hill." Ekerdt's interesting argument is that to fully embrace retirement, Americans have had to imbue leisure with the same connotations of productivity as work.

The Push to Leave Work

Unfortunately, not everyone who retires early leaps happily to embrace the leisure life. "Health problems" are high on the list of reasons retirees give for leaving work early.[11] Figures from the Retirement History Survey underline that people who retire early do tend on average to be less healthy. Early retirees were more likely to visit the hospital in the year before they retired than their co-workers who retired at the normal time.[12]

An underground factor also pushes people to leave work early: age discrimination. Because age discrimination is against the law, it is difficult to prove how prevalent it is among people already working. What can be measured are the variations in hiring rates when older and younger employees are out of work.

Older people are less likely to be rehired after industry layoffs. This is true not just for blue-collar workers but for people looking for high-status jobs.[13] In fact, it typically takes unemployed older workers almost twice as long to find new jobs as people starting out. According to 1984 statistics, whereas job seekers aged twenty to twenty-four were out of work on average for 16 weeks, the mean length of unemployment for people aged fifty-five to sixty-four was 26.2 weeks.[14]

The official unemployment figures for older people are low. But experts agree that these statistics minimize the gravity of the problem because they measure only people actively seeking work. Many older people who are out of work probably get discouraged, abandon the job search, and opt for early retirement. In a recent review, experts estimated that unemployment may be the first step to early retirement for as many as one man in five.[15]

Although we do not have hard statistics on its extent, on-the-job age discrimination is probably not rare either. In fact in a 1978 Harris poll, when employers in a variety of industries were questioned, 87 percent agreed that it was common.[16] Because it is against the law, most discrimination against older workers probably takes a subtle form—not offering an expected raise or promotion, stripping an employee of some responsibilities. When faced with these tactics, many older workers may "voluntarily" choose early retirement to save their pride.

According to Peter Strauss, a New York attorney specializing in legal issues that affect the elderly, the extent of age discrimination in the workplace looks more minor than it is because of the legal system too. The money awarded for winning an age-discrimination suit is small—the few years of salary a worker would have earned by staying on the job until the normal retirement time. So malpractice lawyers tend to be reluctant to take on age-discrimination cases rather than more lucrative ones. A victim of even clear-cut discrimination who consults a lawyer may be advised not to go to court. And retiring a few years early instead of wasting years in litigation often does seem the practical course.

In summary, the legions of early retirees defy categorization. They range from the company president eager for a second career as a skydiver, to the factory hand whose bad back forces retirement, to the manager eased out by having some responsibilities taken away. Because late retirement is much less typical, it tends to attract a more homogeneous crowd.

LATE RETIREMENT

As the early retirement trickle has become a tide, working past age sixty-five has changed from normal to atypical.[17] In 1950 about half of all men worked beyond the traditional retirement age; by 1970 it was one in four; by 1984 only about one in five. (In contrast, since 1950 the small proportion of elderly women workers has dropped only very slightly—from about 10 percent to 7 percent.)

Our attitude toward people who retire late, particularly those who work well into their seventies, is ambivalent. We praise their never-say-die approach, seeing them as models of hearty, involved aging. But we feel squeamish too. There is that nagging question that has dogged our nation's most famous late retiree, President Reagan: "Is he really competent?" And not retiring at the "right" time can also be seen as unfair—hanging on when you should gracefully be making way, depriving a younger person of a job.

Everyone is wondering why at seventy-two I'm still teaching full-time. I have a great pension. I know it's economic folly to stay. But the thought of having nothing to do makes me sick. I am putting off leaving even though I feel like an outcast. Some of the younger faculty act as if I have a bad smell because I'm still here. But even after forty years I adore teaching. I will not give up my life and make way!

A minority of the people who retire late are at the lower rungs of the economic ladder. They cannot financially afford to retire. Many, like this professor, are the educational and socioeconomic cream. They have the freedom *not* to retire and so tend to be self-employed or in jobs having no mandatory retirement age.[18] Almost three-fourths are in white-collar jobs, occupations requiring brains, not brawn. They are usually in one of three fields—service, clerical, or professional/technical.[19]

People who retire late also tend to be healthy, having the stamina to keep working full time. And they stand out in another way: they often dread leaving work. The studies show that workers who hate the thought of retirement are those who buck the tide of early retirement and stay on the job as long as they can.[20] Is their antipathy justified?

The Impact of Retirement

Because retiring is such a dramatic change, even the most enthusiastic person approaching retirement age is anxious: "How will I handle living on a lower budget? How will being retired affect me emotionally? Will I be bored, depressed, and aimless or even die if I don't have a destination from nine to five?" The studies offer reassuring answers to these fears.

THE FINANCIAL IMPACT

Before the early 1970s, retirement had a dire economic effect. In 1960 one out of every three older Americans was poor—a poverty rate twice that of younger adults. Today, mainly owing to improved retirement benefits, older people are no more likely to have incomes below the poverty level than the nation as a whole.

These encouraging statistics obscure the fact that the elderly continue to be significantly worse off economically.[21] Although boosts in Social Security have lifted older people out of poverty, they are still concentrated at the lower end of the economic scale (see fig. 4). In 1984 nearly two in five elderly families had annual incomes below $15,000, compared with fewer than one in five families headed by someone twenty-five to sixty-four years old. And the average income of an elderly family was much less than for a younger family—$18,236 versus $29,292.

Although they do not show its specific impact, these figures

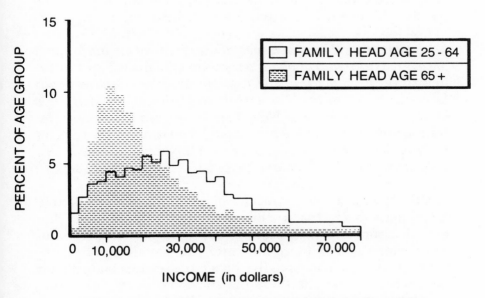

Figure 4   Income distribution of elderly and nonelderly families, 1984

strongly imply that retiring is often a real financial blow. The Duke researchers calculated how heavy this blow actually is. On average people lose 25 percent of their income in the year after leaving work.

Surprisingly, this loss tends to be taken in stride. Most new retirees say their income is adequate to their needs.[22] In fact, in a Harris poll taken in 1981, people under retirement age reported being more bothered by too little income than people over sixty-five.[23] This is not true only of American elderly. In one thirteen-nation survey, the researchers found to their surprise that dissatisfaction with one's "material needs" was at its peak among adults under age twenty-five. In almost every country, the oldest group, people over age fifty, were the most content.[24]

In America, economics partly explains why older people do not feel more financially disadvantaged. The elderly pay a smaller portion of their incomes in taxes than people under sixty-five. They also tend to have more assets and fewer expenses. For instance, three out of four own their homes—80 percent of these "free and clear."[25] Not only are the furniture, silver, and dishes there, but the tremendous expense of raising children is gone. At the same time, special bargains open to "seniors" make it easier to enjoy life's luxuries.

My husband and I bought a special pass from an airline for people over sixty-two. For about a thousand dollars we get unlimited travel for a year. In the past six months we have flown from our home in Fort Lauderdale to California to visit Joe's brother twice. I went to New York for a vacation and to Detroit for my grandson's high-school graduation. After years of scrimping, we are now freer to enjoy our passion for travel. I'm only afraid that I will overdo my jet-setter life and get sick.

Although these compensations help, they do not completely make up for losing a salary. But retirement is different psychologically from any other economic reversal in life. The jolt of being unexpectedly forced to reduce your standard of living is not there. People expect to live on a more limited budget after they retire. Neither is there the sense of having failed that multiplies the pain of living on less—being demoted or fired, investing unwisely, having your business fail. And perhaps most crucial, your retired friends are in the same boat.

Our feeling of not having enough money is surprisingly relative, depending less on our actual income than on how rich or poor we are compared with our friends. Sociologists from the University of Louisville demonstrated this by asking 704 older people whether they were better off or worse off financially than nine people—their three closest friends, closest neighbors, and closest relatives—and then probing their emotional state. How content did they feel?[26]

The researchers discovered that wealth is indeed related to contentment, but wealth as judged by the relative, not real, size of our pocketbooks. If our reference group is millionaires' row, being merely well off is likely to seem a hardship. Being comfortable will feel like being a millionaire if everyone else we know is just scraping by.

Does a smaller pocketbook look more adequate after retirement? A study by John Strate of Wayne State University and Steven Dubnoff of the University of Massachusetts says it does.[27] When a large group of families, varying in income and family size, were asked how much money they would need to "just get along"—the retirees, especially retired couples, felt they needed less than the nonretired families of the same size to make ends meet.

THE PSYCHOLOGICAL AND PHYSICAL IMPACT

The same good news applies to another fear people have about retirement: "I will get depressed and die." It is a myth that retirement is lethal, either physically or emotionally. *The studies show that on average retirement has no demonstrable effect on health or happiness.*

Considering we spend so much of life working, this statistical noneffect on health and happiness seems surprising. However, these findings are averages. Not everyone is affected in the same way. The figures merely show that the people who react negatively to leaving work are canceled out by those for whom retiring is bliss. A more relevant question in looking at your chances for happiness is, Who does well or badly being retired?

YOUR CHANCES OF BEING
A HAPPY RETIRED PERSON

Being healthy and not short of money provides the underpinnings for retirement happiness. Not unexpectedly, retirement smiles on people who are not ill and who have the financial resources to enjoy life.[28]

Apart from these background factors, your attitude is important. People who are very unwilling to retire not only leave work later, but also are more unhappy once they take the step.[29] On the other hand, looking forward to retiring predicts positive things. So one key to judging what will happen after retirement is to trust your instincts about how you will feel.

Some nervousness about the future is normal no matter how positive your feelings are. To judge whether your fears have merit, ask yourself these things: "Do I have absorbing hobbies or exciting ideas for how to spend my time?" "Do I love being with people?" If you answer yes to each of these questions, you are likely to be a satisfied retiree. However, some very sociable people do find retirement a deprivation if by leaving work they cut out a good chunk of their social lives.

We tend to carry ourselves with us as we shed our work skins. So look carefully at your personality. Are you a happy, well-adjusted, positive person? If so, you are likely to be a happy, well-adjusted retiree. And look at how you live your life now for a projection of your retirement life-style.

In one of the early retirement studies, sociologists found male retirees fit into five personality types; three were adjusting well, and two were handling retirement poorly.[30] The types were:

1. The "mature man": This type of person looked at the world and life realistically, was not upset about growing older, and saw life as fulfilling. His mature attitude toward living made for a happy retirement life. (Luckily, most of the retirees in this study fit into this category.)
2. The "rocking-chair man": This type of person disliked responsibility, preferring to take a backseat. Because retirement allowed him to indulge this need, he too was happy being retired.
3. The "armored man": Keeping extremely busy was im-

portant to this type of person. The idea of contemplating his navel—or his feelings—made him very anxious. Surprisingly, he too was likely to be a happy retiree because this gung-ho advocate of the busyness ethic frantically packed his leisure day with activities.

The people who were unhappy were the "angry men"—those who felt they had been failures and bitterly blamed the world—and the self-haters. The latter also were unhappy about how their lives had gone but blamed themselves.

With the exception of the mature men, many of whom said they had grown emotionally as the years passed, these men seemed to be the same people as retirees as they had always been. The angry men and the self-haters had been unhappy and badly adjusted in youth and middle age. The armored men and rocking-chair men had approached their working years in the same way they handled retirement.

So while we can look forward to retirement as a chance to fulfill our basic nature, we cannot expect it to make that nature basically different. Though the words (or content) of our new lives may indeed be dissimilar, the melody or basic style we live by is likely to remain the same. But on the way to finding the retirement melody that fits us, we may strike some sour notes.

THE ADJUSTMENT PROCESS

Retirement expert Robert Atchley believes people go through stages before finding the right retirement niche. Immediately after leaving work, there is a honeymoon period when everything is rosy. People either luxuriate in doing nothing or excitedly pack in leisure activities. Then a letdown sets in. Something is missing. Either people do too much and end up exhausted, or they begin to feel at loose ends without anything productive to do. At this point there is an evaluation phase: "How do I really want the rest of my life to go?" After this period of reflection, most people are able to evolve a satisfying retirement life.

Though these phases are idealized and theoretical, a study by David Ekerdt, Raymond Bosse, and Sue Levkoff supports their general outlines.[31] When they interviewed 293 men at varying points after leaving work, these researchers did find high levels of optimism, happiness, and activity in the first six retirement months, followed by a letdown at the beginning of the second year. Just as Atchley predicts, after the first excitement phase, disenchantment does seem to set in. Luckily this study also bears out his optimistic prediction that most people will emerge from this slump. Although the heady feelings of the first months never reappeared, among people approaching the two-year mark after retirement happiness and activity levels were higher again.

Planning for Retirement

The studies show that if you have a generally good feeling about retiring, reasonably good health, and enough money— and most important, are basically a happy person—you are likely to be happy as a retiree. Planning will also help. Not only will it ease your anxiety, it will help you avoid the blind alleys and disenchantment that sometimes characterize the second retirement year. Go in with the right attitude: "I am not being put out to pasture. These are the years to reap my rewards. I must not squander the rest of my life. I plan to make these decades the most fulfilling I can!"

ECONOMIC CONSIDERATIONS

Take comfort from the fact that living on a lower retirement budget is often easier than people expect. But also take these steps before you retire:

Write down how much income you will have as a retired person. Consider your income from savings, from your pension, from Social Security, and from any other source. If you have the choice of several pension plans, choose wisely. Be clear about the differing types of coverage, eligibility, and spousal/dependents benefits offered by each. Understand the tax status of your benefits.

Estimate the value of your assets. Knowing the value of what you have in reserve is important for your peace of mind.

How much could you expect to get from your investments, your home, and your personal property if an emergency occurred and you had to convert your assets to cash? (Get professional help from an accountant or your bank in making this assessment.)

Estimate your expenses. Then turn to the other side of the ledger. Determine how much it is likely to cost (or now costs) you each month to live. Consider all expenses—rent, mortgage payment, insurance, taxes, loans to be repaid. Estimate your utility and grocery bills and the amount you are likely to need for such things as clothing, transportation, medical and personal care, household supplies, repairs, travel, and entertainment.

If your calculations show you have money to spare, great! If you end up on the debit side, come up with some livable strategies for reducing what will be going out. Or would you feel comfortable selling some assets in order to live?

Give living within your retirement income a trial run. Live as a retired person for a few weeks. If this exercise suggests that your budget will be uncomfortably tight and dipping into capital is out of the question, at least you know. Now is the time to stay on your job a little longer or perhaps begin to look for other work.

EMOTIONAL CONSIDERATIONS

Because the psychological side of life cannot be captured in numbers, planning emotionally for retirement may seem more difficult. Not so! Taking these steps may help you come up with concrete solutions for the aspects of retirement you fear. (Adapt these suggestions to help get yourself on the right track if you are already retired and at loose ends.)

Imagine your life as a retiree. Think about what an average day or week would be like. What kinds of things would you do? Is your general mood upbeat, or can you only imagine being depressed? If you cannot imagine being happy, consider this a very important warning light. Trust your gut feeling and try to put off leaving work as long as you can. If you know you will have to retire in a few months, start exploring new job possibilities. It is much easier to get a new job while you are still in an old one. You will be less frantic, and potential employers are likely to feel you are more desirable if you approach them having a job in hand.

Pinpoint your exact concerns. If you are like most people, you can imagine being happy but have a sense of foreboding too. Focus on exactly what concerns you, and if necessary write each worry down.

Come up with antidotes for each worry. Then brainstorm, drawing up battle plans for eliminating your concerns. Preferably, come up with a few possible solutions to each problem you foresee. For instance, your list of anxieties and antidotes might look like this.

Worry 1: I'm afraid of the lack of structure. How would I plan my day from nine to five? I can just imagine that listless feeling if the highlight of my morning became waiting for the mail. It would be terrible to wake up with each day stretching out as a soul-destroying monochromatic blank.

Solutions: Before I leave work I will have some sort of structure in place. I'll sign up for a course at the local university. I'll arrange to go swimming at the gym every day. I'll go to a senior citizens' center—the one that is open every day. I resolve never to go to bed with absolutely nothing planned for the next day. I will have at least one destination in place for tomorrow before I turn out the light. But I won't overdo it. This is my time to enjoy smelling the flowers. It would be a shame if, out of anxiety at being aimless, I frantically rushed around.

Worry 2: I'm afraid I would miss my work friends. I can just see myself hanging around the office the way Joe did after he retired. I remember how foolish he looked, arriving at eleven for those lunch dates at one o'clock.

Solutions: I'll join a club; cultivate that person I always liked who works across the hall and is retiring now too; avoid the office but keep in contact with my work friends at night and on weekends.

Worry 3: I'm afraid no longer being an important lawyer will depress me deeply. I can just imagine myself cringing inside when I go to a cocktail party and someone asks me what I do. I get such a kick out of telling them I'm a partner in Thomas and Belsky. It will be terrible to say I'm retired. I care so much about the status and satisfaction I get from work; my drive to accomplish something and be a productive professional is such an important part of who I am.

Solutions: To people who ask I will say, "I retired in 1988 from Thomas and Belsky." More important, I have to find something else that gives me the same boost I got from work.

A person is likely to feel that work is irreplaceable when it seems the only way of satisfying some basic human needs— pride in achievement, the joy of showing what you can do. Your goal is not to damp down these needs or to live with frustration, but to have retirement fulfill them too.

A whole industry has sprung up to gratify the need to feel creative, competent, and useful that does not end at age sixty or ninety-five. But you have to stop equating being productive with being gainfully employed. If you get hooked on knowing about the world (e.g., traveling or reading), or collecting antiques, or even on a sport like golf, you will find the same pride in stretching your capacities that you once felt was possible only through work. The truth is that "the busyness ethic" discussed earlier is not just a hook that gets people to leave work. It is genuinely important to our happiness as human beings to feel that what we do at any time of life has meaning and purpose. Aimless retirement is as soul-destroying as aimless work.

Settle on a life that will really engross you. To help yourself, use the techniques outlined in chapter 3. Consider your best qualities, the aspects of yourself you prize most: for example, "intellectual," "friend," "civic-minded person." Then select retirement activities that will capitalize as much as possible on these qualities. As the research in chapter 3 suggests, fitting your retirement life-style to your "identities" is a good way to help ensure that your life will be happy—that your days will have purpose and meaning. Then consider the hobbies, interests, and activities you enjoyed in the past—if necessary, decade by decade from adolescence to now. Pay special attention to ambitions, goals, and hopes that you may have had to put aside. This is the time of life for fulfilling abandoned dreams.

In my law school class, I ranked third. My fellow students have been judges and senators, and at least one is a Supreme

Court justice. But I was forced into the family bedspread business soon after graduation. From the first I disliked the work and knew I was no good at the job. A few years ago when I was sixty, the business that had suffered for years under my bad management went bankrupt, and I was forced to retire. Jane and I moved to Saint Petersburg and lived a modest but comfortable life. At first I was happy just to golf and fish and enjoy not working, but after about a year I got bored. I got the idea (though I had not practiced in over thirty years) of returning to law. I studied for months, took the "impossible" Florida bar exam, and passed. I got a job at a small firm. The pay is not great, but I am finally doing just what I really want. And I am a great help to the firm. After years of feeling terrible about myself, I have an elegant new identity—that dapper older partner from Yale.

If you are not sure what direction to pursue and are interested in finding yourself in a more systematic way, professional help is available. Specialists in career counseling—helping people plan their work lives—have expanded their skills to a new area called leisure counseling, planning a fulfilling *postwork* life. A leisure counselor will give you tests to assess your preferences and will help you formulate your goals. The placement service of your local college (community colleges are best) may offer information about leisure counselors. Or look in the Yellow Pages under career or vocational counseling. Some of the employment services listed in the section on job seeking in the Epilogue may also do leisure counseling.

Your self-analysis may lead you to decide to return to work at least part time. And despite the existence of age discrimination, the employment rate after retirement is surprisingly high. One-quarter to one-third of all people reenter the work force at least for a time after they retire.[32] Or you may choose a gratifying job as a volunteer; take advantage of the low-cost opportunities to get a college degree; fulfill a lifelong interest in the arts. In putting any of these dreams into action being older is an advantage, because special opportunities are open to you. (Turn to the Epilogue for a discussion of these options.)

As a vital retiree you are a tremendous national resource.

Understand your value and make the most of these precious years. Rather than your being out to pasture, marked for imminent death, retirement is the time when full and free living becomes most possible, and so potentially the most gratifying time of life.

For More Information

ABOUT AGE DISCRIMINATION IN EMPLOYMENT

American Association of Retired Persons. *The Age Discrimination in Employment Act Guarantees You Certain Rights. Do You Know Them?* and *The Age Discrimination in Employment Act Protects Your Rights. Here's How.* Washington, D.C.: AARP, 1985.

Write to the American Association of Retired Persons' Fulfillment Section, 1909 K Street N.W., Washington, D.C. 20049, for free copies of these brochures explaining the Age Discrimination in Employment Act, your rights, and your remedies if you feel you have been discriminated against on the basis of age.

Equal Employment Opportunity Commission, 2401 E Street N.W., Washington, D.C. 20507 (202) 634-1947.

The place to write for information and to file charges if you are a victim of age discrimination.

BOOKS

Palmore, E., B. Birchett, G. G. Fillenbaum, L. K. George, and L. M. Wallman. *Retirement: Causes and Consequences.* New York: Springer, 1985.

This is the Duke University research I drew on so heavily in this chapter. It gives an overview of the reasons Americans retire and the consequences of retirement by examining the most comprehensive studies in the area. Scholarly.

CHAPTER

7

WIDOWHOOD

My husband was treated with medication for angina, but the pain went from bad to worse. Then he went for an angiogram. Knowing the test is dangerous, I was terrified he would die that day. Then came relief: it was over, and he was still alive! Now that we knew what was wrong, I was sure the right treatment could be started. The children and I almost danced into Dr. Eagen's office to get the results.

The verdict was short. "The heart muscle is severely damaged. Nothing we can do will help. Joe is terminally ill. He could die tomorrow. With luck, he could last a few months." I was surprised at the way I took the news. I did not even want to cry. I felt clammy and distant—observing life.

Often during the additional six months Joe did survive, I had the same eerie sense of being emotionally disconnected from what was happening. We never discussed things. We both knew he was dying but went on as if everything had not totally changed. Tom, Sara, and I measured time by the holidays Joe survived. He lived through Easter and our anniversary in May. He made it to Tom's law school graduation but was so weak he could barely stand up. In September, the end came. That morning, looking at the exhausted shell he had become, I thought: "I can't stand this waiting much longer. When will you finally die?"

These first two years as a widow have been hard. A few weeks after the funeral the feelings really hit; frightening dreams, terror at sleeping or eating alone, the sense of being cut off. No one, not even the children, really understood my pain. I saw Joe turning the corner, felt his shadow in the room.

And I hated him—for not saying good-bye or helping me prepare for life on my own.

Within the past few months I think I've turned a corner. I've gotten a job; I'm doing well. I still hate being alone in our king-sized bed. I think about him ten times a day. But one feeling I never thought would reappear is there: I am beginning to enjoy living again.

The death of a spouse hits with a double blow. It means not just the loss of a life companion but the end of a whole way of life. Jobs that may have seemed impossible—untangling the finances, cooking meals, fixing the faucet—suddenly fall on the new widow or widower. Even waking up takes on new meaning when it is done alone. Other people may be lost along with one's spouse. Friendships can be changed and sometimes broken, for many close relationships during marriage are based on being a couple. Other ties may weaken or erode—relationships with in-laws, the other side of the family.

As British psychiatrist Colin Parkes, an authority on bereavement, explains, widowhood has to produce this dramatic ripple effect. Being married is like being female or Catholic or smart, a fact through which we filter and interpret our other experiences. When our identity as a married person is gone, our perceptions of everything else alter too: "Even when words remain the same, their meaning changes. The family is no longer the same object it was. Neither is home or a marriage."[1]

People can be unprepared for the magnitude of this change. Ignorant of the sometimes strange symptoms of normal bereavement, they may think they are going crazy. They may wonder when they will feel better or be shocked at the cold or angry way they feel toward relatives and friends. They may be astonished at how different they have become: social butterflies may turn introverted, introverts may be incapable of spending a second alone. They may also question whether they are doing right: "Would it be better to stay alone with my thoughts or go out?" "Am I a terrible person not to want to see my married friends?" "Should I move or stay in this house full of memories of him?"

More Widows,
Many Fewer Widowers

This ignorance about what to expect is particularly unfortunate for women, because their chances of being widowed are so high. Of the approximately 12 million widowed people in the United States, about 10 million are women;[2] because women now outlive men by 7.4 years, the differences in numbers are especially striking at the oldest ages. For instance, in 1984 two out of three women over age seventy-five were widows, a figure exactly reversed for the opposite sex: two out of three men still had living wives.

This difference in longevity plus the fact that most women marry older men is also making widowhood a distinct era of life. Not only will many women spend their last years as widows, but the average widow will survive her husband for about fifteen years.[3] Here is how the numbers affected one new widower.

When I was young I had fantasies of being pursued by women; I wondered what it would feel like to be propositioned, to sit back and be chased. Now I know. Since Alice's funeral, I have barely had time to think, much less to mourn. I took a vacation with my daughter in part to keep the invitations away. Someone even had the nerve to propose to me while Alice lay dying. It was one of her best friends!

While not all widowers are besieged like this, older men do have an easier time finding women. And it is generally believed that they are much more likely than widows to jump into the arms of a new mate. But how firmly are older women locked into widowhood compared with older men?

In the mid-1970s, researchers at the University of Southern California got some fascinating indications by examining nationwide marriage rates for 1970 for men and women over sixty-five.[4] Although the probability that an older person of either sex would marry during this twelve-month period was small, it was indeed much smaller for women than men. Whereas seventeen out of every thousand older men married that year, women had fewer than three chances per thousand of walking down the aisle. Furthermore, that year's elderly grooms were not choosing wives from among their age-mates. A full 20 percent had brides younger than fifty-five.

In the same year, researchers at Duke University answered a similar question: At various ages, what are the chances of remarriage for widows versus widowers?[5] Comparing North Carolina marriage and death records, they discovered that men and women widowed before age thirty-five have a very high probability of remarrying—chances that decrease steadily for both sexes at older and older ages. But the decline is much steeper for women than for men. For instance, by age sixty-five to seventy-four white widowers have about one chance in four of remarrying; the odds for white widows are a meager .004 percent.

Do Older Widows Want to Rewed?

These odds seem just fine for many older widows. They often say they do not want to marry again. They are indelibly bound to one man; they would never find husbands as good as their dead mates. Some are afraid remarrying will mean being a full-time nurse; in a study of 301 Chicago widows over age fifty, one-sixth had nursed a husband at home for at least a year before his death.[6] Widows may all too accurately weigh the chances of a repeat performance when a potential suitor appears.

Last week I got a marriage proposal but didn't give saying yes a second thought. The man was an old friend and attractive, but he is eighty years old! At age seventy-six I'm not so well myself. When he proposed, images of nursing Sam flashed before me. I am lonely and I like him, but what would I need that aggravation for! I think widowers are more needy than me or my widowed friends. We can give them a good deal. What really can they offer us!

Do men need marriage more than women do? Information on how each sex adapts to widowhood implies that they may. Though the studies do conflict, a recent review of the literature suggests that if there is a sex difference, it is men who tend to cope more poorly with a spouse's death.[7] There also is a male/female difference in the time of highest risk. Men seem most vulnerable to severe emotional and physical problems right after their loss. Women are more likely to develop the worst difficulties in the second or third year. Particularly, *older* women tend to handle the trauma of bereavement best; of anyone, they are least at risk for becoming ill.

For instance, the saying about long-lasting marriages, "Soon after one goes the other does," may have a grain of truth—but only for men. When Duke University epidemiologists examined mortality rates among several thousand North Carolina residents for several years after they were widowed, they found that though widows did not have a higher death rate, the death rate for widowers was elevated and stayed that way. A widower's chances of dying dropped to normal for a man his age under one condition: if he remarried.[8] One explanation for this fascinating finding is that widowers who are healthier to begin with selectively have the energy (and desirability) to find new mates. Another, more interesting interpretation is the one women have always surmised: marriage itself is good for a man's health.

These statistical differences are small. And some recent very careful studies comparing just elderly widows and widowers have not found gender differences in how people react.[9] Actually, whether we are male or female is not the issue. If sex differences in adjustment do exist, they are relevant only because they offer insights into what *is* important in helping us cope. What is it that might make men more vulnerable than women to losing a spouse?

As I described in chapter 3, close relationships seem to offer us emotional insulation, cushioning us from breaking down under stress. Men tend to have fewer genuinely intimate relationships than women; when their wives die, they often lose their only confidants. So one reason women may cope better with this terrible stress is that they tend to enter widowhood with their eggs in more than one emotional basket.

A study of 351 older people done by University of Texas psychologist Neil Krause underlines how important this type of widowhood insurance may be.[10] When Krause looked at how effective close relationships were at warding off depression in the face of different traumatic events, he found that, more than for any other crisis, supportive friends and family were important in preventing depression after the loss of a spouse.

Friends, even more than family, may be good widowhood insurance,[11] as sociologist Helena Lopata first discovered about twenty years ago when she did an in-depth study of more than three hundred Chicago-area widows over age fifty.[12] Because of Chicago's insulated ethnic neighborhoods, the women in her landmark study of widows were ethnically and economically diverse and also differed greatly in how thoroughly assimilated (Americanized) they were. Most were well past the rocky period of adjustment, having been widows an average of eleven years.

Because their lives had focused narrowly on their families, the "Old World," least-assimilated women were having the worst problems coping. Having just their children to fall back on for comfort after their husbands' deaths, they were often disappointed. They expected more than they were likely to get. Many were bitter. They wanted life the way it used to be. Their children, no matter how loving, had gone on to make new lives. But the more middle-class, Americanized widows were doing better. They had not wrapped themselves in a cocoon during their married life. Because their lives were richer before they became widows, their husbands' deaths did not rob them of absolutely everything.

But if having choices and opportunities is so important, why do older women, who seem to have the least chance to make a new life, cope so well with losing a spouse? Once again, one reason may be friends.

When a woman is widowed in her twenties or thirties, where does she turn? Her friends are newlyweds or new parents. They cannot understand what she is going through. Fate has singled her out for an arbitrary blow. An older woman who loses her husband feels just as bereft, but she has been to other funerals. Though she may not realize it, she is better prepared mentally for being a widow. At the funeral of a friend's husband the thought, "That could be Tom," may have crossed her mind. (Her husband sitting next to her may have a feeling that ill prepares him for being widowed: "That could be me!")

When her husband does die, her feelings are just as sharp, but they are less unexpected and less frightening because they have a reference point: "what Mary went through in those dreadful first days."

This unconscious comparison, forced on older women by the statistics, may be very helpful. Having the path marked out allows the grieving widow to focus on her loss without fearing for her sanity. It can help her understand that there is light at the end of the tunnel. Eventually people do adjust. But are widows (and when they have the chance, widowers) right to judge their emotions by the yardstick of friends? When we lose a husband or wife, can we *expect* to feel certain ways?

Normal Bereavement

The first scientific attempt to chart mourning grew out of a famous disaster, the Coconut Grove fire that took the lives of several hundred people in Boston in 1942. The following year Erich Lindemann, a young psychiatrist at Massachusetts General Hospital, interviewed people who had lost loved ones in the tragedy.[13] This study and a study of the emotions of London-area widows during the first year of bereavement are classics, showing that mourning does follow a predictable course.

Losing a loved one is similar to a severe physical wound. The pain is unbearable at the beginning, then gradually subsides. As the wound heals, there may be days when the agony is nearly forgotten and others when it reappears almost full force. Although people differ in how long the healing takes, sooner or later recovery generally is complete. A scar remains, but the person is able to resume a full life.

Yet some injuries never heal properly. The wound still festers; the pain never goes away. The same applies to losing a husband or wife; some people never recover emotionally. Even years after their loss they remain immersed in mourning and feel incapable of going on.[14]

WHAT IT MEANS TO RECOVER FROM BEREAVEMENT

Although we never fully "forget" a loved one's death, normally after some time people are able to think about their loss without intense pain. The memory no longer has the same wrenching quality. The reality of the death has penetrated, and an adjustment has been made to a new life. In the early months a widower may have half expected his wife to walk through the door; now he knows in his heart she is dead. Instead of spending hours crying, incapable of doing anything, three years later a widow fills her day with friends or her new job. Though the pangs of grief still well up sometimes and special times such as birthdays and holidays may always be bittersweet, the widowed person is able to live and love again.

More formally, bereavement expert William Worden of Harvard University says mourning involves four tasks.[15]

Accepting the reality of the death. Right after someone dies, there is usually a sense that it hasn't really happened. People understand the facts intellectually but still feel that at any moment they will wake up from a bad dream. The first job of mourning, which normally takes place during the first few months, is to believe in the truth emotionally.

The rituals surrounding the death start this process. Being forced to deal with the practical circumstances of the burial teaches a new widow or widower that functioning is possible. And it helps reality begin to penetrate: "My husband (or wife) is actually gone." The service, the burial, the reception exist not just to honor the deceased, but to certify to the survivors that the death is real. Because they serve this reality-inducing function, Denman Dewey, director of the gerontology program at Marymount Manhattan College in New York, advises that the more the newly widowed person can be involved in the practical arrangements surrounding the death, the better. Every action taken helps bring home what has happened and so helps in the eventual adjustment to a new life.

Queen Victoria is a legendary example of a person who never got past this first step. Decades after the death of her consort, Prince Albert, she still had fresh clothes laid out for him daily and often went around the palace speaking to him. Because she never absorbed the fact that her husband had died, for her the role of new widow became a life career.

After two years do you still see your dead wife on the street? Are you still setting your husband's place at the dinner table even though he died five years ago? These are some signs of not having accepted the reality of death.

Feeling the intense pain of grief. Because cultural and individual expressions of grief vary enormously, mourning deeply does not have to mean weeping or wailing; it may mean retreating, dry eyed, to a quiet place to think. But it does mean confronting your feelings directly. Many experts feel that pain sidestepped is only postponed.[16]

After six months are you amazed at how little you feel about your husband's death? Rather than missing your wife, do you have a host of physical complaints? Does it seem as though your spouse's death was "nothing at all" in spite of your close, thirty-five-year marriage? Is your only emotion relief? Sailing right through a trauma of this magnitude may mean rough emotional waters later on.

Adjusting to a new life. This task takes longer to complete than the first two. During the first few years after being widowed, people learn to be competent in areas their spouses had taken over. They gradually make a new life.

Can you list many ways you have changed and grown since your wife's death a year ago? Do you feel more at ease (even if not happy) about being on your own? Are you venturing out in the world again? These are some signs of grappling successfully with the job of remaking your life.

Loving other people. Worden cautions that this task can present particular problems for widows and widowers. People cut themselves off from other relationships because of guilt, the idea that by loving again they are being disloyal to their husband or wife. If you feel any new relationship would debase what you had, take this cliché to heart: One sign of a loving marriage is being able to love again.

Although it is not necessary to want a new romantic involvement, it is important to regain the capacity to love in a broader sense. To know if you are recovering in this crucial area, ask yourself: "Do I care about people and things again?"

HOW LONG SHOULD THESE TASKS TAKE?

Though the most intense grieving occurs during the first year, according to Worden accomplishing these tasks often takes as long as two years. Other studies suggest that, particularly for widows, three years may not be too long.[17]

Putting a timetable on bereavement is difficult. How can we fix a date for finishing mourning when many people say they never completely get over their spouses' deaths? So use these tasks as general guidelines, keeping Worden's words in mind: "Asking when mourning is finished is a little like asking how high is up."

Another problem with using these benchmarks is that they wrongly imply that grieving gets less intense in a linear way— that as time passes people just feel better and better. Actually, the intensity of a person's feelings and the ability to cope normally fluctuate.[18] For instance, some people may have what is called "a six-month reaction." After they have handled things remarkably well during the first few months, raw grief suddenly wells up. At the beginning the widowed person is in a daze, with life taken over by relatives and friends. When the invitations slack off, the reality of the loss hits.

A minor event may set off intense grief. A widow may completely break down when she struggles to put up the storm windows the first October after her husband has died. A widower may suddenly feel bereft when he has to do the Christmas shopping alone.[19]

When researchers at the University of Utah charted widows' and widowers' feelings at regular times during the first two years of bereavement, they discovered just how great an oversimplification it is to expect people to feel better and better as the months pass. The words "better" and "worse" do not capture the complex, chaotic, often conflicting feelings that wash over people as they struggle to come to terms with their loss. A good example was in the tumultuous first months. At that time scores on tests of *both* depression and self-esteem were very high. In other words, rather than just feeling "awful" at the beginning, people felt a mixture of emotions, both very upset and also very proud about the way they were handling things. And while it was true that over time these intense feelings subsided and people did gradually make a new life, even as the two-year point approached they sometimes had flashbacks of feelings characteristic of the first shocking days and weeks—disbelief, avoidance of the truth.

THE FIRST SYMPTOMS OF BEREAVEMENT

How do people act and feel during those intensely disorienting first weeks? A poignant description comes from an ethologist, not an observer of human grief—Konrad Lorenz's observations of a greylag goose that had lost its mate.

> The first response to the disappearance of the partner consists in the anxious attempt to find him again. The goose moves about restlessly by day and night, flying great distances and visiting places where the partner might be found, uttering all the time the penetrating trisyllabic call. . . . The searching expeditions are extended further and further and quite often the searcher gets lost, or succumbs to an accident. . . . All the objective, observable characteristics of the goose's behavior on losing its mate are roughly identical with human grief.[20]

One early symptom of bereavement is searching. The widow or widower symbolically acts out the drive to be reunited so beautifully described by Lorenz. A woman may see her husband's face in a crowd; feel him hovering just out of sight. For many new widows and widowers, the impulse to search becomes a compulsion to go over and over the events surrounding the death, as if by rewinding the tape of what happened in the last hours and days a different ending can be forced to magically appear.

The first month I would wake up at 4:00 A.M. and review again and again what happened in the hours just before. Tom was having slight chest pains, but we weren't too concerned. The doctor told him to check into the hospital, but we took our time getting there; we managed to get stuck in rush-hour traffic. Suddenly, on the highway, I heard a gagging sound, and my husband slumped down in his seat. We couldn't find the police to flag down, and by the time we got to the hospital it was too late. I kept asking myself: Why? Why didn't we rush to get out? Why didn't we call an ambulance? Why was the traffic so heavy? Why was Doctor Jones so nonchalant? I imagined how just one element could be changed and it could have added up to his still being here. It was almost as if I could

*make things turn out differently by repeating every twist of
the terrible chain of events.*

Because these preoccupations are so strange, they can make
the newly widowed person feel that he or she is going mad.
But they may be normal and instinctive, both in people and in
animals. According to British psychiatrist and ethologist John
Bowlby,[21] they are a manifestation of our inborn, lifelong reaction to separation, seen most clearly in infancy when a baby
clings, cries, and crawls vigorously after his mother when she
leaves the room. Bowlby believes that the loss of our "primary
attachment figure" (first parents, later husband or wife) instinctively calls forth a similar "attachment response" at any
time of life—we try frantically to be reunited at all costs.

New widows or widowers may also feel guilty, regretting
every marital lapse: "Why wasn't I more understanding?"
"Why did we argue that morning?" They may take personal
responsibility for wielding the ax: "I should have insisted he
give up that stressful job." "If we had moved to Florida the
way she wanted, she might not have had a heart attack."

People may become irrationally angry, blowing up at children and friends. Even the dead spouse may not escape their
rage: "Why didn't he prepare me better for life on my own?"
"Why didn't she take better care of her health?" When people
are hurt they tend to lash out—blaming the world, blaming
themselves. But this reaction can boomerang. When a widowed person turns against friends and relatives, it may cause
them to run away. They may be frightened into retreating just
when their support is needed most. Anger turned against oneself or one's husband or wife adds a dose of guilt to the burden
of the loss itself. Not only does one lose the loved one, one
loses self-esteem.

Another target of (sometimes) misplaced anger is doctors
and "medical science." We expect doctors to be the restorers
of life, and we get angry when they fail—blaming their proçe-
dures, their techniques, and their decisions: "The chemother-
apy that was supposed to help just prolonged his suffering."
"That operation shortened her life." Above all, we blame

them if their bedside manner is bad; sometimes with good reason.

Can you sue a doctor for emotional malpractice? That's what I feel like doing. Henry was a powerful business executive. When he put on his hospital gown, Dr. Zaccarelli commented: "Isn't it funny how an important man looks just like any nobody without his clothes?" When we visited his office and Henry complained about constipation or another side effect of the medicine, this healer looked mockingly past my husband and winked at me. He seemed bent on diminishing my husband, turning him into a nonperson because he was going to die—blaming him for being sick!

While mild anger and self-blame are not unusual symptoms of bereavement, when these emotions are intense or overshadow all others, they may be a sign of pathology. Psychologists James Breckenridge, Dolores Gallagher, Larry Thompson, and James Peterson interviewed 196 older men and women two months after their spouses died.[22] The participants in this study of early bereavement were mainly well educated, middle class, and long married, having been wed an average of thirty-seven years.

Only 25 percent reported feeling guilty; fewer than 10 percent felt intensely angry at anyone. The most frequent symptoms people did have were continual crying, extreme sadness, and problems with sleeping and eating.

According to the researchers, the absence of intense anger and self-blame may differentiate mourning that is normal from mourning that is pathological—in which the widowed person is developing a clinical depression that needs treatment. People suffering from depression usually feel "terrible about myself and the world." These emotions, when present to a marked degree in a new widow or widower, suggest that mourning is not progressing normally—that the widowed person is becoming depressed and may need psychological help. Among the many influences that may predispose people to develop this type of pathological bereavement response, here are a few possibilities.[23]

Excessive experiences with death. In some ways, previous

deaths of loved ones should help us cope with widowhood. We know what it feels like to mourn; we know we have handled things in the past. However, too many losses may create a kind of emotional overload, depleting us psychologically and making adjusting to the present loss more difficult.

Emotional immaturity. Not only are poorly adjusted people less able to handle stress, our past reactions to stressful events may offer clues to the way we will deal with widowhood. Are you good at handling the worst? When devastating things happened before, what exactly did you do? You can get some idea of how you will react to this loss by looking at how you reacted to tragic events in the past.

An untimely death. A loss that seems particularly unfair causes special pain. If your husband dies right after the retirement he slaved for, your grief is likely to be more intense than if he dies in his nineties after living for years in a nursing home. If your marriage was just beginning to click, being widowed may be more difficult to bear than if you had fifty wonderful years.

The quality of your marriage. Not all marriages are the same. How strongly being widowed affects us is related to the strength of our attachment to what is lost. However, having had an excellent marriage may actually make recovery easier. In studying a large group of widows and widowers (granted, under age forty-six) during the first year of bereavement, Harvard University psychiatrists found that people with unhealthy marriages—those who were extremely dependent on their spouses and those who were often on the verge of divorce—were at higher risk of suffering severe, unremitting bereavement responses.[24]

Anyone who has a happy marriage is dependent. We open our hearts to need when we open them to love. But needing someone is very different from rushing into another's arms out of fear. The people in this study who were rated as having dependent marriages used the relationship as a refuge from the world. Rather than a platform for full living, marriage was a cocoon for avoiding life. Unless they could find someone else to lean on after being widowed, they remained immersed in mourning—incapable of building a new life.

This makes sense, but why would an unhappy, conflict-ridden marriage produce a more rocky, prolonged bereavement? Wouldn't losing someone you really loved produce a more yawning emotional gap? This description from my aunt, Frances Sheerr, offers clues.

I married Stanley when we were young. We were together for more than forty years. I still miss him terribly, but I'm getting along. He taught me to feel strongly that what you give is what you get. Because we were fulfilled in each other, we could be generous. It was important to him to be affectionate and considerate, to tell me continually how wonderful I was. I naturally found myself doing the same with other people I cared about. Throughout this year my friends have stuck close. My children value my company and want me around. And because our marriage was so good, I miss him terribly but am not eaten up by regret. The happiness we found in each other offered me a legacy crucial to withstanding this tragedy: loving children and caring friends.

Because it strengthens us as people, a loving marriage may paradoxically help us remake an independent life after a husband or wife dies. And because love is infectious, a happy marriage may leave us richer in confidants to soften the blow. However, someone who loses a spouse who was more devil than saint enters widowhood weakened and battle scarred. The marriage was far from wonderful; death may even bring a feeling of liberation. At the same time, seeing the marriage as having meaning may be important to achieving closure and going on. But the widowed person remains stymied by the truth, perhaps wracked with resentment and guilt about these feelings. The intense anger and guilt spell depression—a pathological mourning response.

When loved ones die there is a natural impulse to award them a halo, epitomized by the injunction "Don't speak ill of the dead." While the difficulty of doing this causes problems for survivors of unhappy marriages, it can compound grieving after the most loving unions too. For instance, a man may have adored his wife for her gentle spirit but hated the way she always left the house a mess. After her death he may seethe with self-hate when he feels relieved at walking into a clean house. But he is wrong in feeling that his emotion is "bad" or that it subtracts from the love that was there. No human being is an angel. The best memorial to someone we love lies in remembering the real person who lived.

Some Practical Advice

Although the research is most relevant to widows and widowers, it also offers lessons for married people and anyone who is close to someone recently widowed.

FOR MARRIED PEOPLE

The main message for married people boils down to the standard advice: Preparation helps! Emotional preparation is particularly important. Don't depend on your immediate family for everything in your life. While you are married, try to develop other interests and, in particular, at least a few friends. Understand, even though you naturally feel closest to your children, that they have their own lives. There is danger in entering widowhood with the expectation of depending just on a son's or daughter's visit or call.

Particularly if you are an older married woman, you are being prudent, not ghoulish, to plan ahead. If you are a man, planning is even more important because you are at higher risk for coping poorly. Don't push the thought "my husband (or wife) could die" out of your mind. Mentally take stock of how you would manage in case the worst did occur. Imagine your daily life. Who would you depend on for company and support? Would there be satisfying things you could do other than "being with my mate?" If your answers are unsatisfying, cultivate a more independent life now.

Consider practical issues. Women in particular *must* know whether they will be provided for financially. Don't stick your head in the sand and then discover to your horror when your husband dies that your savings are minimal and his pension doesn't cover you. Ask and insist on being let in on his financial arrangements for you and the family, and educate yourself in the particulars of the family finances now.

Men too can benefit from educating themselves in the practical side of being alone. Become competent at shopping, cooking, and cleaning, and if you have not already done so, periodically give your wife a rest by taking over these jobs. Not only will you be preparing for being widowed (and possibly learning some interesting new skills), you will be making your wife feel appreciated and loved.

This brings up another essential way of preparing for this blow. Make sure that if your husband or wife died tomorrow you would not be eaten up by guilt about what you did not do. Demonstrate your love now!

FOR FRIENDS AND RELATIVES

You are likely to feel awkward, wanting to be helpful but not knowing what will help. It is a rare person who isn't nervous about expressing condolences, who doesn't hate confronting a new widow or widower. Most of us recoil at dealing with strong emotions. Even if we feel that speaking about what has happened is best, it is hard to see crying without taking action to gloss over the hurt. Yet words are so inadequate. The knee-jerk response is to resort to platitudes that sound silly even as they tumble from our mouths: "Think how lucky you were to have those wonderful fifty years." "Time heals everything."

Experts advise that often the best thing to do is say "I'm sorry" and then listen—to give the widowed person a chance to talk.[25] Your goal is not to make things better; nothing you say really can. Respect the person's need to open up, but do not force the issue. Respect his or her dignity too.

Keeping occupied has saved my life during these six months. My friends and family have rallied around and are careful not to let me spend a long time by myself. By "being kept busy" I do not mean running away from thoughts of Stanley and the beautiful life we had. Almost every day my daughter Jane calls and we cry together: "Poor Daddy. Why did he have to suffer so!" I like being with friends who knew and loved us as a couple. We can share memories, and I'm not ashamed to cry. On the other hand, I hate being forced to emote when I don't want to. This happens most often with acquaintances who think they are being helpful by probing my inner state. The other day I was humiliated to find myself breaking down at the dentist's. He had asked the question I think widows must hate most: "What a terrible tragedy! How are you getting along?"

Widows and widowers are touchy. Even when you try your hardest to be sensitive, you may feel you are putting your foot in your mouth. But it doesn't matter. Develop a thick skin and hang in there. Even if you are rebuffed at times, what is important is that you continue to be there. We tend to remember the people who stick by us in adversity. Now is your chance to become—or ensure that you stay—treasured in the life of someone you care about.

Although advising the widowed person on practical matters that you have special knowledge about (such as the burial or taxes) may be helpful, avoid advising on matters of opinion: "You should be going out more." "Why don't you sell your house?" Try to restrain yourself when the impulse strikes to intervene in this way. Remember, it is understanding—not advice—that people need most. When you feel like making a suggestion, decide to ask this question instead: "What can I do to help?"

You may need to extend your mental timetable for how long things should take. Do not expect someone to have "recovered" after a few months. On the other hand, if more than a year has gone by and absolutely nothing has changed, then step in. You have a responsibility, to put it delicately, to tell your relative or friend that something is wrong: "People are usually not this distraught for this long. Perhaps you might want to think about getting professional help."

FOR WIDOWS AND WIDOWERS

Although knowing the research will not ease your suffering, use it to ease your anxiety. If you have strange or frightening sensations they are probably normal, not signs you are going crazy or breaking down. (The exception is strong fantasies of hurting yourself or someone else physically. Then you *must* get professional help.)

Confidants help. Feel free to lean on as many people as you can. If being alone is very difficult, call someone. But be selective—call someone who will make you feel better, not worse. If you want help with specific things, ask. If you genuinely would prefer to be alone, don't be too polite to refuse invitations. Let people in on what you need. Give others the chance to be helpful by not forcing them to read your mind.

If you focused your whole life on your husband or wife, don't let my emphasis on the importance of planning depress you. Most of us are more resilient emotionally than we think. And even when people enter widowhood with everything against them, they often adjust remarkably well.

Don't have unrealistic expectations about what you should be feeling or when you will be your old self again. Understand that getting back to "relatively normal" can take as long as a few years. Don't be disappointed if you seem to be getting better one month and the next are overcome by grief. It is not normal to just improve and improve. Everyone takes two steps forward and one back. If possible, plan for the days you know will be difficult: birthdays, your anniversary, Christmas. Would having a friend over help? In the past, what strategies have gotten you through difficult times? Feeling especially vulnerable on special occasions is normal; it would be shocking if nature made us so malleable that we could completely forget.

Make the thirteenth month a time to assess your progress. How were you at the beginning compared with now? What can you do today that you couldn't do a year ago? In what concrete ways has your pain lessened? You might list what you have accomplished: "doing the taxes; eating in a restaurant alone; stopped crying every night." And since you may have trouble being objective, ask your family and friends: "How do I seem now compared with the first few months? Do you see signs that I am getting over Jack's death?"

Most likely, making this assessment will boost your morale. You will realize you are indeed better in many ways, even though you are far from being over your loss. But if it does not, knowing this is important too. Do you still think about your husband twenty-four hours a day? Are your eyes just as red rimmed and about to brim over? Do you feel just as incapable of loving? Are you still wracked by guilt? If more than a year has passed and all of you still seems to have died along with your spouse, consider getting professional help.

Expect some lack of understanding from others. People may get angry because it is more than six months later and you are not reciprocating for all those dinners. They may not realize you still feel too disorganized even to cook for yourself. They may feel hurt because you would rather be alone than go out. You may meet the opposite type of censure: "How dare he insult Mother's memory by marrying so quickly?" "It's appalling the way she goes out with different men all the time!"

Friends and family may also pressure you to do things or make decisions, feeling strongly (but wrongly) that it is best not to "dwell on things." Out of their natural urge to do something helpful, they may advocate your taking all sorts of concrete actions: selling your house, moving to Florida.

Although ultimately making dramatic changes may be important in building a new life, experts recommend not undertaking any radical life changes during the first six months.[26] People in the midst of grieving are not in a good position to decide how their lives should go. And being widowed itself is a tremendous change; piling on more changes will multiply the stress.

During the first year, take most advice about how you should behave with a grain of salt. There is no single best way to act. The way you are feeling and acting is likely to be best for you. If you prefer to be alone, don't capitulate to a friend who urges you to keep busier or get out more. Your next friend is likely to counsel, "It's better to be by yourself to think." Neither judgment is necessarily right. At the same time, don't get angry at friends and relatives. You need their support. Educate them.

Try to cultivate at least one sympathetic widowed friend. Talking to another person who has gone through what you are dealing with can be a great relief. And coming from someone who has been there, the platitude "things will get easier" is not empty. It carries real weight.

Widowed Persons' Groups

Strongly consider joining a widowed persons' group, even if you have an abundance of friends and are not the joining type. During the past few decades widowed persons' services have become widespread, sponsored by community centers, associations for the elderly, and religious organizations. There is a reason for their popularity. In dealing with this type of wrenching loss, people need all the help they can get.

Your local office for the aging will have information about these programs. So will the Widowed Persons' Service operated by the American Association of Retired Persons (see the end of this chapter). Or look in the Yellow Pages under "widows" or "widowed persons' services." The most logical place to begin your search for a group is a place you already feel comfortable going, such as your church.

Generally, widowed persons' services either offer individual counseling in which a trained (less recently widowed) volunteer visits you regularly or operate groups where widows and widowers meet to discuss their feelings and offer each other concrete help and emotional support.

Widowed persons' groups are for normal people, not those who are emotionally disturbed. They offer a place where you can feel comfortable about expressing all your concerns—from the fear of going crazy to "silly" worries such as "How do I make coffee?" or "How do I check into a hotel?" Attending a group can also offer more subtle benefits.

Because I am a private person, I hated to tell my friends and relatives how out of control and lost I felt. There were so many practical things I needed to know: how to manage the money, how to deal with my mother-in-law, how to tell my children tactfully that they were treating me like a child. The widows' group was a perfect solution. Even though not everyone there was just like me, our meetings gave me the chance to compare. Best of all, I was transformed from "poor Mrs. Johnson

who needs sympathy" to "Mrs. Johnson who is able to reach
out to others in need." Once I found myself being helpful to
other group members, I knew I would make it. I realized I
could help myself too.

Consult as many books on widowhood as you can. There are
now guides to handling problems ranging from the most prag-
matic (dealing with the funeral director, paying estate taxes)
to the most abstract (getting through the day). Anyone who
has been widowed should consider the information in this
chapter a starting point. Visit your library or bookstore. There
are so many things to educate yourself about!

This tragedy does have a silver lining. It is a chance to experience the love of family and friends and a chance to know
yourself. In spite of their difficulties, many of Lopata's Chicago widows said their husbands' deaths had taught them an
important lesson. They were stronger and more capable than
they had ever thought.

For More Information

ABOUT WIDOWED PERSONS' SERVICES

AARP Widowed Persons' Service, 1909 K Street N.W., Washington,
D.C. 20049　(202) 728-4370.
Provides programs for widowed persons; offers a telephone referral
service to local widows' groups. Call for information about widowed persons' services in your area.

National Association of Military Widows, 4023 25th Road North,
Arlington, Virginia 22207　(703) 527-4565.
Offers widows' services to military widows.
(Also check your local church or synagogue, office for the aging, or
Yellow Pages for widowed persons' services and groups.)

SCIENTIFICALLY ORIENTED BOOKS

Lopata, H. Z. *Widowhood in an American City.* Cambridge, Mass.:
Schenkman, 1973; and idem, *Women as Widows: Support Systems.* New York: Elsevier/North-Holland, 1979.
Lopata's studies of the lives of the Chicago Widows. Aimed at a
professional audience, but also interesting for the layperson.

Parkes, C. M. *Bereavement: Studies of Grief in Adult Life.* New York: International Universities Press, 1972.

Beautifully written scientific account of the first year of mourning.

Parkes, C. M., and R. S. Weiss. *Recovery from Bereavement.* New York: Basic Books, 1983.

Once again a moving, beautifully written description of the authors' research on the first year of widowhood, this time among a group of Boston-area men and women widowed before age forty-six.

PRACTICAL SELF-HELP BOOKS

Bozarth-Campbell, A. *Life Is Goodbye/Life Is Hello: Grieving Well through All Kinds of Loss.* Minneapolis: Comp Care, 1982.

How to deal with grief.

Brockman, E. S. *Widower.* New York: Bantam, 1987.

The first book to explore the plight of the widower. A daughter writes feelingly about her father's experiences as he struggled to cope with being widowed.

Grollman, E. *Concerning Death: A Practical Guide for the Living.* Boston: Beacon, 1974.

Covers the practical aspects of death—funeral, condolences, and so on.

Peterson, J. *On Being Alone: AARP Guide for Widowed Persons.* Washington, D.C.: AARP Widowed Persons' Service, 1980.

Free brochure offering guidance to the newly widowed (write to the AARP, Box 199, Long Beach, California 90801).

Wylie, B. J. *The Survival Guide for Widows.* New York: Ballantine, 1982.

Comprehensive guide to the practical problems of widowhood.

(The Widowed Persons' Service of the AARP also publishes a current bibliography.)

CHAPTER

8

LIVING ARRANGEMENTS AND CHANGING RESIDENCE

I want to move to see my grandchildren grow up, to enjoy their development firsthand, not by phoned progress reports. Even though Philadelphia is not far from Providence, our visits are frustratingly infrequent—and just as often, uncomfortably intense. We must plan for months to find the rare weekend everyone has free. We stay at my daughter's house, and we get on each other's nerves. I long to just drop in and take the girls for an hour or so. I hope I would be more help than burden. As a doting grandmother and a reliable backup caretaker, I could relieve the pressure Sarah is under, the times she must get to work and the baby-sitter calls in sick. I also want to move because of me. At age sixty-nine a day will come when I will need her help. Why not go now, when Joe and I are healthy and can make new friends? The longer we wait, the harder it will be.

My husband is lukewarm. We have lived here for twenty-five years and have made a life for ourselves. We don't know anyone in Providence. He thinks I am dreaming about making new friends at my age. The house is way too big, but selling it would be like getting a divorce. Every corner is a part of us. We don't have to sell to make ends meet. Would we really feel at home in a small apartment in an unfamiliar town? What if we do turn out to be a burden? Will my daughter resent us? Will I be able to avoid intruding in her life? Would my other daughter be hurt that I was choosing her older sister, not moving to Chicago to be near her? The idea of the New England winters bothers me—Could they really be that different from the cold down here last year? I'm doomed to go back and forth until Joe retires and we make a decision. I wish I knew the right choice.

Many of us link retirement with the thought of moving, especially if we live in the North or Midwest. As we buck the cold or fight the rush-hour traffic, we may dream about taking life easy in Florida or Arizona during our retirement years. But when retirement day finally arrives, how many of us translate this dream into action, taking our pensions, packing up, and fleeing to the Sunbelt?[1]

Some of us do. Although the proportion of older people increased somewhat from 1970 to 1980 in each state, it rose most dramatically in the Sunbelt. Furthermore, of the 1,662,520 Americans over age sixty who migrated out of their home states during this decade, nearly half went to five states, four of which are in the South: Florida, California, Arizona, Texas, and New Jersey.

Florida lives up to its reputation as our nation's top retirement destination, in the past two decades capturing more than one in four migrants over age sixty. And as we all assume, it does have a much higher percentage of elderly residents than any other state. Whereas in 1984 people over sixty-five made up 12 percent of the total United States population, 17.6 percent of all Floridians were over this age.

On the other hand, the retirement exodus is highly overrated. If people fled south after retirement with real frequency, by now we would have a bottom-heavy country, with the highest concentration of older people in the Sunbelt. We do not.

Apart from Florida, the states with the highest proportion of older residents are not in the Sunbelt. Arkansas, Rhode Island, Iowa, Pennsylvania, Missouri, South Dakota, Massachusetts, Nebraska, Kansas, Maine, and West Virginia all have an elderly population of between 13 and 14 percent. And in 1984 older people joined the rest of the nation in living primarily in our nation's eight most populous states, five of which are in the North or Midwest: California, New York, Florida, Pennsylvania, Texas, Illinois, Ohio, and Michigan.

Migration and Reverse Migration

Who does migrate? Charles Longino offers some clues by charting the flow of older people into and out of particular states over the past few decades.[2] This University of Miami demographer calls Florida a migration "winner" because older people who move there from other parts of the country are mainly younger (in their sixties), more affluent, and healthy. Migrants from Florida to other states (usually northern or midwestern ones) are likely to be older (over age seventy-five), poorer, and more in need of nursing-home care or help with living independently.

California is a "winner" or "loser" depending on the state it is being compared with. It gains in exchange with Illinois, because older migrants from Illinois to California are better off than people who migrate in the opposite direction. But because Arizona has replaced California as a destination for young, well-off retirees, California now "loses" in comparison with its neighbor to the southwest.

The comparisons made by Longino and his colleagues show there are fashions in retirement locations. By analyzing migration patterns from 1960 to 1980, they find that Florida, Arizona, and Texas are becoming more attractive as retirement destinations, while the lure of once very desirable California and New Jersey has waned. More important, their figures show that today there are *two* types of retirement moves: the well-known exodus to the "hot" (literally and figuratively) retirement states made by more youthful, fairly well-off people just after retirement, and a smaller, less-noticed reverse migration years later. Some retirees who moved "forever" to a Sunbelt state in their sixties are forced to return to their home states in their eighties when they become physically frail, have trouble living by themselves, and need their families near.[3] There can come a time when people are "too old" to stay in their retirement homes.

Not Moving—the Norm

Most older people do not move even once, however. In spite of their reputation as migrants, people over sixty-five are the least likely to change residence of adults of any age.[4] Our early twenties, not our sixties, are the time of life when we are most likely to move. As the years pass and we establish roots in a place, we are increasingly likely to stay put. For instance, while more than a third of all twenty- to twenty-four-year-olds (and about a fifth of the nation as a whole) changed residence from 1982 to 1983, only about five out of every hundred people over sixty-five moved that year.

The strong resistance to moving that characterizes many older people is suggested by another demographic fact. Apart from Florida, the counties with the highest concentration of older residents are in rural areas in our nation's heartland (see fig. 5). Whereas younger people living in these often economically depressed counties have left in droves for more urban areas, the older people refused to move. And when the elderly do move, they tend to resettle within their area; moving to a new community or state is rarer.

A survey sponsored by the American Association of Retired Persons offers other clues to this stability. Why are most older people so wedded to where they are? What type of housing are older Americans likely to have, and what are the pluses and minuses about where they live?[5] In the fall of 1982 the AARP commissioned a polling organization to conduct telephone interviews with a nationwide sample of more than a thousand Americans over age fifty-five. The poll showed that people stay in one place not out of fear or lack of money but because they like living where they are. Most people rated their housing as good or excellent. It scored the highest points on comfort and location. The most frequent complaint people had was the lack of good public transportation.

Not unexpectedly, more affluent people were likely to give their housing high ratings. People who felt safe (not afraid of

1980

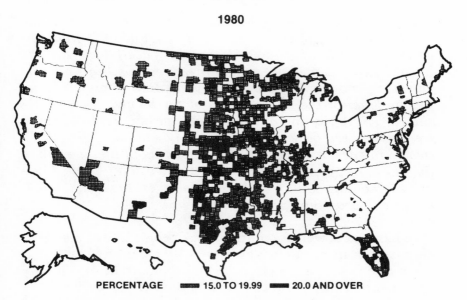

PERCENTAGE ▬▬ 15.0 TO 19.99 ▬▬ 20.0 AND OVER

Figure 5   Counties with 15 percent or more elderly residents, 1980

crime), those who were in good health, and—surprisingly—
those who lived in large versus small cities (presumably because public transportation in large cities tends to be good)
were also especially pleased with where they lived.

The poll suggested that as we get older we vote no to moving
because our roots are too deep to be casually pulled up. The
vast majority of the people surveyed owned their homes
(about 80 percent). More than half had been living there a long
time, at least ten years. The largest fraction, 39 percent, had
lived where they were from twenty years to a lifetime.

When we live in one place for so long, our home becomes
part of us. It is more than an asset to be traded away. So even
though it may seem logical to move to a smaller space, or to a
place where life is easier, we hesitate. Our home is so thick
with memories that leaving can be like cutting off our past.

*I live in a beautiful four-bedroom house in the suburbs. John
and I bought the land and had it built when we were in our
thirties, in the first blush of his business success. The house
was a symbol that we had made it, that we didn't have to*

struggle anymore. We resisted the impulse to sell when the children went off to college and everyone told us it would be better to live closer to town. After John's death last year, the logic to leave seemed overwhelming. So far my heart has prevailed. By moving I would lose my last link to my husband. Every corner of the house is full of the happy moments we shared. The dining room still reminds me of those lovely family dinners; the backyard is where my son and husband retreated to have man-to-man discussions about life. In spite of the effort in upkeep and my isolation, I don't think I can move. And how could I trade the beauty of this scenery for a sterile one-bedroom apartment in town?

Economics as well as emotions lock people in. For instance, because rent increases in New York City are limited by law, it is not rare to see widows living hand-to-mouth in large luxury apartments. Although the space and the exclusive address far from affordable shopping are more of a burden than a gift, these women cannot afford to give up the 1950 prices and leave.

Moving also becomes less of a compelling idea when people calculate the cost of living in their homes versus apartments. For most of us a home is our primary asset. Eighty percent of homeowners over age sixty own their homes free and clear. So particularly in states that offer older people a reduction in property taxes, an older homeowner's living expenses are small. The price Mrs. Jones's home would bring on the market may seem dazzling, but what happens after she sells? The alternatives—exorbitant rent, a high purchase price and monthly assessment for a condominium—may seem worse than what she has now—space, memories, the yard, the luxury of not shelling out a hefty monthly check.

And even when they are financially able to move and want to do so in theory, people do not move because they are afraid: "What will happen if the choice is wrong?" "Isn't the stress of changing likely to be too much for me at my age?" Especially moves to places known as old-age destinations can be fraught with ghoulish symbolism: "People retire to Florida to die." "If I give up my home for Century Village I will age just by proximity, being around all those 'old' people." Are any of these fears realistic?

The Effect of Moving
on Physical and Mental Health

When we say Mr. Smith's heart attack was caused by the stress of retirement, blame our brother's death on his anguish over being widowed, or nod ruefully when we catch the flu the week we move, we are agreeing to a belief as old as ancient times: that major disruptions in the pattern of life make people sick. For most of this century, however, this idea was pooh-poohed by a medical profession bent on explaining illness in purely medical terms: "Physical diseases have physical causes. Except for a very few stress-related conditions (e.g., ulcers), our emotions have no effect on how our bodies behave." In the late 1960s, Thomas Holmes and Robert Rahe decided that rather than simply accepting the unquestioned dogma, they would actually test the "old wives' tale" that stressful events can make us ill.

They assigned change rankings to a list of events, scores ranging from a high of one hundred for being widowed to lows in the teens for minor upsets such as getting a traffic ticket. Because they felt that the sheer quantity of change itself, not whether the change is bad or good, produces illness, they included both negative and positive events on what became their well-known life-change scale (see table 4). After testing thousands of subjects, Holmes and Rahe proved that there was indeed a nonspecific link between outer-world changes and internal ones. People who had unusually high change scores during a short period were more likely to get sick. Depending on their particular vulnerabilities, they were more susceptible to illnesses as varied as cancer and colds.

Not everyone who retires, moves to Florida, and loses his wife in 1988 is fated for a hospital bill—or even a cold—in 1989. People vary greatly in their physical stamina and in their capacity to absorb and tolerate change. Events also have very different meanings for different people. As we saw in chapter

Table 4   Some Items from the Life-Change Scale

Life Event	Change Units
Death of spouse	100
Divorce	73
Marital separation	65
Death of close family member	63
Getting married	50
Being fired	47
Reconciliation in marriage	45
Retirement	45
Pregnancy	40
New member in family	39
Change in finances	38
Death of close friend	37
Change in work responsibilities	29
Moving	20
Minor law violation	11

Source: Adapted from E. K. Gunderson and R. Rahe, Life Stress and Illness (Springfield, Ill.: Charles C Thomas, 1974).

6, for instance, it is not true that the man who hates his job is affected in the same way by leaving work as his friend for whom retirement is a catastrophe.

In fact, contrary to what Holmes and Rahe predict, a recent study suggests that happy events may not be illness producing at all. Researchers at Indiana University School of Medicine questioned elderly residents of a public housing complex about their health, then compared their answers with the total number of changes versus the number of negative changes they had recently undergone. Only the *negative* events tally was related to declining health, suggesting that it really is our new misfortunes—not our new blessings—that affect our physical well-being.[6]

So we need not fear the physical consequences of moving. Change in itself does not seem to be bad. However, we do need to ensure that moving will be a positive change in our life. Does the research offer any guidelines in making this judgment? Yes, if we examine research on moving to nursing homes.

After moving to a nursing home, many people deteriorate mentally and physically. But some improve. People are likely to do well after entering a nursing home under two conditions: if the place they move to is a step up from their life outside, and if their personalities fit the requirements of nursing-home life.

If we are impoverished, in very bad health, and live an isolated life, going to a nursing home is likely to boost our health and well-being.[7] Being there is an improvement from the terror of trying to cope outside. Researchers find that people who are tough, assertive, and insensitive are also likely to do well in nursing homes because they have qualities that uniquely suit them for institutional living.[8] Their talent for fighting gets them more of the limited resources available. Their harder-than-normal hearts help insulate them from the suffering around.

Luckily, the personality that equips us for success is very different in less harsh places. However, the criteria for judging whether we will do well are the same: Is the place you are going better or worse than the one you are coming from? Does your new home fit the kind of person you are?

For example, when gerontologist Frances Carp compared older people who had moved into a retirement residence—a high-rise building with a community center—with another group who had applied for the housing but stayed in their own homes, she discovered that, instead of being worse off, the people who moved were happier and healthier.[9] Even though they were somewhat less involved with their families, they had more friends and were more active and involved in life than the nonmovers.

One reason was that the retirement residence was indeed a better place than most of these low-income elderly were coming from. Not only was it physically more appealing, it offered a safer, socially richer life. But living in the residence was not good for everyone. Some people were unhappy after they moved. Introverts had particular trouble; they disliked the greater social pressure to get involved in their new home. Their preferred style of living—to keep to themselves—did not fit the togetherness ethic at the residence, so they felt alien, uncomfortable, and unhappy after they moved. In other words, apart from whether it is better objectively, you must judge whether the place you are considering fits *you* emotionally.

In a 1985 follow-up to this study, Carp went back to the residence to find out what personality traits predict happiness in housing of this type.[10] She found that people who were congenial, extraverted, and well adjusted were flourishing—content with themselves, popular with the staff and residents. So housing for older people is far from being all alike. The personal qualities that suit us for living in an unhappy place (a nursing home) and a happy one (this retirement residence) are totally opposite.

For the older people Carp studied, the move to the residence was a step up. Often there is no obvious difference in quality between retirement housing and what people can buy or rent outside. So studies show that residents of retirement communities are on average as satisfied or happy as people who remain (or live) in traditional homes. There also is no evidence that living in a retirement community decreases health problems or health complaints. But people who live in retirement housing, particularly places that have many programs, do tend to be more active socially. They are more involved in groups and leisure activities than the average person their age.[11]

So the studies show that you will not die sooner (or live longer) by moving to a retirement community; and even though you may emerge a bit from your cocoon, neither will you shed a lifetime of shyness and become a social butterfly. We take ourselves with us wherever we go. But since having the chance to live in this type of housing is such an interesting new opportunity that being older offers, retirement communities deserve a closer look.

Retirement Communities

A retirement community is a self-contained complex for people over a certain age. However, this description says nothing about the variety that exists among the estimated 2,300 that have sprung up in every corner of America since the end of World War II.[12] They are popular. About a million people are currently choosing the retirement community life.

A retirement community may be an entire new town or subdivision. Or it can be a high-rise building. It may be in the middle of a forest or be a converted landmark in the center of town. It may range in size from a small mobile-home park to Sun City, Arizona, with its 45,000 residents. A variety of housing designs and arrangements are available as well as a variety of agreements regarding financial and living commitments. Some communities offer a full range of recreational and educational activities—golf, tennis, indoor and outdoor pools, classes, a clubhouse. Others provide varying levels of personal and medical care. Or a retirement community may be nothing more than a housing development restricted to people past a certain age. There are even retirement communities with no age restrictions at all.

For instance, the Greens at Leisure World,[13] in Silver Spring, Maryland, is typical of a large recreation-oriented retirement complex. A variety of activities is available—a pool, tennis courts, golfing, exercise and card rooms, lectures, and classes and groups of different types. While the additional cost is very small, most of these amenities are not included in the monthly maintenance residents pay. Homes here are relatively expensive, making the Greens primarily for upper-middle-class people (one spouse must be over fifty). Unlike its more isolated counterparts in Florida or Arizona, this retirement community is close to Washington, D.C. It has single-family homes, apartments, and semidetached units.

The Greens provides no paid-for medical care or meals (though there is a medical building near the grounds). Goodwin House, in Alexandria, Virginia,[14] and Otterbein Home, in Lebanon, Ohio,[15] typify housing for people who want to live in a place that includes more personal services and health care.

At Goodwin House (a single building) residents buy their apartments and then pay a substantial monthly fee. Their payment includes meals, personal and nursing care, and maid service, plus educational and recreational activities. At Otterbein Home the facilities are spread out more and differentiated by what are called levels of care. There are three types of independent housing—duplex apartments, cottages, and low-rise apartment buildings. In addition there are three levels of health care—personal, intermediate, and skilled (the last two are classifications of nursing-home care). Contracts involve an entrance fee and monthly payments, with a resident either paying for everything in a lump sum at entrance and each month or paying extra when more medical or nursing care is needed. Goodwin House and Otterbein Home exemplify the most innovative type of retirement community—the continuing-care or life-care community.

ADVANTAGES

As the popularity of retirement communities shows, they have some distinct advantages over traditional housing.

They offer a relatively worry-free life. Being planned with older people's needs in mind, retirement community living tends to be more convenient, easier, more anxiety free. Often essential services are nearby or on the grounds—food store, pharmacy, bank. If not, good transportation is available. Communities tend to have excellent security systems, minimizing the fear of crime. Residents are also more protected in case of a medical emergency, even if their community does not offer health care. Many complexes have an emergency call service. Some pay for their own ambulances to ensure residents immediate attention in a medical crisis.

They help prevent loneliness. Retirement communities can substitute for the social function a job or school had earlier in life. They are places where making friends is easier. Even if a person is not interested in the activities or the courses, the pool, clubhouse, and dining room (if your contract includes meals) are easy meeting places. And since everyone is a relative newcomer, residents tend to be more open to new friendships.

This makes a retirement community a good place to consider if you are moving to a new area "cold." If the warmth of Florida is enticing but you hesitate about migrating because you don't have friends there and meeting new people at your age seems too hard, a retirement community may offer a warm social climate to complement the weather in starting a new life. Or if you are moving across the country to be near your children, by buying in a local retirement community you might not have to feel so fearful about burdening your son or daughter with the job of providing all your social life.

They promote a healthful life-style. Retirement communities tend to be health oriented, making them good choices if being (or becoming) physically fit is a priority in your life. Health clubs, lectures on preventive medicine, exercise classes, and outdoor activities are staples of many communities. Retirement-community dwellers tend to be physically aware and committed.

When I was visiting my friend at Green Acres, I looked out the window at 7:00 A.M. and saw hundreds of people walking briskly around. In addition to exercise machines, classes, tennis, and the pool, the residents had organized this morning walk! I thought of the trouble I have just leaving my Chicago apartment at that hour—cold, fear of getting mugged—and how foolish I would feel if I jogged or exposed myself to the Yuppies in that exercise class at the Y (getting there is a half-hour ride on the bus). I love the city, but it set me thinking. If I move here, I might live longer; at home the whole thrust is toward dying. It's such an effort to do anything!

DISADVANTAGES

Living in a retirement community is not for everyone. You may like diversity and chafe under the sameness of seeing only people your own age. You may feel isolated from your roots if you move to a community far away. You may find the cost prohibitive. Many communities are for people of financial means. Many are also outside urban areas. Would you miss the stimulation only a city can provide? And there are other problems basic to living in this type of housing.

You lose some freedom of action. By living in a retirement community, you frequently give up some latitude in determining your life. You may have to pay for services you do not use. You must abide by the set of rules the community lays down. You may have a good deal of say in how restrictive these rules are, or you may not (see the discussion below). Sometimes the most unpleasant restriction is the most ele-

mental one: no younger people allowed. What would happen
in a family crisis if your daughter and the baby needed to move
in?

You lose some anonymity. Particularly in a small community where meals and communal activities are offered, it may
be hard to keep to yourself. As in any place where everyone
knows everyone else, there may be social pressures to get involved. If you are a private person, you may find the push to be
friendly and join group activities constraining. You might prefer living in a more impersonal place, where you are not vulnerable to Mrs. Jones's invitations whenever you walk out
your door.

Your future may not be that anxiety free. If you have moved
far from your family and medical care is not provided at the
community, what would you do if your health deteriorated
and you needed your family near? Would you have to move
back to your home state? If you are in a rural community,
what would happen if you could no longer drive? Some people
find that the whole character of life changes when they are isolated by a minor disability that prevents driving. Even regular
bus service and a city minutes away do not prevent the sensation of being cut off.

Because health problems can unravel this way of living that
people choose for its stability, evaluate any potential retirement community with regard to both your present and your
future needs. Shop for your ideal now and imagine the worst.
Would I have to move if I could no longer live independently?
Ideally, there should be a hospital or nursing home nearby.
The layout of the community should make getting around easier (e.g., there should be ramps and no steep steps).

If your needs do change and you have to move, make sure
getting out will not be too difficult. How much of your investment would be refunded if you decided to leave? How easy
would it be to sell your home, given that you must sell to another retiree?

There can also be financial anxieties attached to *staying* in a
retirement community:

*When I bought my apartment here in 1978, the pool, the golf
course, and the health club were free, and my maintenance
was a hundred dollars a month. Now all the amenities are ex-*

tra and my monthly charges have increased fourfold. So far I can afford things, but I worry about the future. One of my neighbors had to move because she could not afford the increases.

Although at the time you buy your home it may be hard to predict exactly how much your future costs will rise, you can get an idea by examining the current financial health of the community you are considering. Ask for documents such as the annual report or financial statements and discuss them with a qualified person—perhaps a banker or an accountant. Learn who sponsors or owns the community and what their financial responsibility is. Assess whether the management seems to have the experience to run the community well. As I will describe in the next section, getting a full picture of a prospective community's financial health is especially critical if you are moving to a continuing-care retirement community.

A fascinating study of thirty-six representative retirement communities conducted by a research team at the University of Florida in the early 1980s underlines that people who choose this type of housing may have more worries than they bargained for.[16] The researchers classified the communities they studied into two ownership types. In type 1 communities, the residents own the land the community is on. Once the developer withdraws, they are responsible for running it. In type 2 communities, the residents rent the land from the owner/developer, and so the community's fate continues to be in outside hands.

Living in each type of community entailed special anxieties. In type 2 communities, where the developers stay boss, the residents were vulnerable to their decisions. For instance, an owner might raise the rent drastically, impose new community rules, or even sell the community to another person who might change its character totally by renting to younger people. In the type 2 communities the research team studied, residents usually passively submitted to developers' decisions because they were afraid of what might happen if they made waves. They were particularly concerned about the ace in the hole their developers had if they made too much trouble: selling the community to someone else.

The worries of residents of type 1 communities centered on

their own ability to govern themselves. What if competing resident factions vying for leadership polarized and fragmented the whole community? Or as a community and its residents grew older, what if no one wanted to assume the job of governing? This is not to say the residents were miserable or felt they had made a mistake. But they were a bit disappointed. Living in a retirement community was less like heaven and had more real-world risks than they had imagined.

CONTINUING-CARE RETIREMENT COMMUNITIES

In most retirement communities the focus is on recreation, not health care. While housekeeping or an optional meal may be available, residents are on their own and may have to move if they need help living independently.

Continuing-care or life-care communities are different. Medical and nursing services are the most important part of the package. People choose this type of community for the security of knowing they will have a place to live and the services they need (provided they keep up their monthly payments) if they do become disabled or need nursing-home care.

As Laurence Branch of Harvard Medical School explained in a 1987 article, at the core of the continuing-care concept is nursing-home insurance.[17] People have banded together in a self-insurance group so they will not be left penniless by going to a nursing home. All continuing-care retirement communities offer some nursing-home care, though they differ in how extensive this coverage is. Because of their health-care focus, they also usually offer more services for people with minor disabilities than a traditional retirement community would— maid service, three meals a day, help with bathing and dressing.

Because so much more is included, a considerable financial investment is often required. Though arrangements differ, in most communities residents pay a large fee when they enter and monthly payments after that. Still, if the costs are added up, a person is likely to spend considerably less than if the services were purchased individually.

As is true of any type of housing, continuing-care communities vary in character, price, quality, and services. In some places residents have the option of paying for all services at the beginning or of paying for them as they are needed. Life expectancy is also a factor in computing a prospective resident's fee.

There tend to be health restrictions to admission. Communities want their residents to arrive relatively healthy, so many require a physical examination. If a person fails the screening, the community generally refunds the deposit minus an application fee.

The obvious advantage of living in a continuing-care community is peace of mind. Not only are you insured (at least in part) against catastrophic illness and severe disability, but you know where you will go and the exact quality of the services you will be offered if you need protective or nursing-home care.

These advantages are offset by some definite negatives. For instance, the package deal is an even more severe limitation on choice. In continuing-care contracts many unused services are apt to be included in your bill—meals, transportation, possibly even the nursing home. And your security still depends on being able to keep up with your monthly costs. What was once paid "for life" may be extra a year later; your monthly fees may rise dramatically. There are horror stories of bankruptcies and the risk of losing everything you put in. So before investing in this type of arrangement, use extreme caution. Go in with your eyes open about everything financial that applies to the community you are considering.

According to Branch, the economic risks of continuing care are threefold: enough people have to buy into the community at its beginning stages to keep it afloat; enough healthy new residents must enter subsequently to keep costs within reasonable bounds; and the expense of caring for ill residents must not become prohibitive.

In a 1986 seminar on the problems of life-care communities, experts explained that this last condition—being in the business of providing health care for life—is what makes continuing-care retirement communities so financially vulnerable.[18] No one can predict how much health-care costs will rise. It is also surprisingly hard to know how much in the way of services a given group of life-care residents will need. Actuarial statistics are used to compute the community's probable health needs, leaving its residents vulnerable if an unexpected proportion of their number are very ill. If the illness odds go against a community, residents may have two unpleasant alternatives: a steep rise in their costs or bankruptcy. As of late 1987 there is no federal legislation to protect the life savings of people who invest in continuing care. A 1986 national survey showed that only twenty states had passed protective laws.[19] So, though unlikely, it is possible to lose your nest egg if the worst occurs.

Because there is statistical safety in numbers, the speakers at the seminar sponsored by the National Council on the Aging urged that people interested in continuing care buy into a large community, preferably one owned by an established corporation or company. Small communities sponsored by unknown developers should be avoided.

In addition to investigating its financial health, before entering you must know if you will like what you are paying for. Visit several times, thoroughly checking out a prospective community's quality and services. Use the American Association of Homes for the Aging checklist on pages 206–7 to ensure that you are not missing anything (see table 5).[20]

Suggestions for Making Any Type of Move

In making any move, whether to a continuing-care retirement community or not, the research suggests you should take these additional steps.

List the pluses and minuses of your new home versus your current one. Compare objective dimensions such as cost, convenience, and beauty, and concentrate on intangibles too: "Knowing myself, is this place likely to bring out the best in me?" "With my interests and needs, would I be content living here?"

Be as clear-eyed as you can about your new home. If fleeing south to avoid the harsh northern winters seems so appealing, consider how you would cope during sweltering summer days. Visit for a week in August before you leap to pack up. If an apartment seems desirable because maintaining your house is so hard, think how it would be to lose the space, or the memories, or to pay rent each month. Balance realistically the joy of moving to be nearer your family with the pain of being parted from old friends. Be very cautious about moving for motivations like "watching the grandchildren grow up." Your family may love you dearly, but their main life must be apart from you. Be reasonably confident that you will be able to make a satisfying new life apart from them in your new home.

Consider your future health. What would life be like here versus there if it becomes more of an effort to walk or drive? Your new home (ideally) should be within a few blocks of essential places—the bank, the drugstore, the grocery. Or transportation should be good and very close by. What physical barriers will you have to negotiate to get out of the house? Those stately steep steps and that lovely quality of being set back from the street might become nightmarish if they make you housebound because of a minor disability. In weighing the virtues of moving, keep accessibility—and access to good health care—in mind.

If your decision is to go, the research on life change offers some guidelines to planning the move.

Move during a peaceful time in your life. Minimize the risk of getting sick by not moving at a time when you are dealing with other major life changes. Don't move to Florida the week you retire—wait a few months. Particularly if you are moving to a totally unfamiliar place, keep your agenda clear of simultaneous adjustments that will add to your stress.

Set up as much as possible of your new life beforehand. Lower the change value of the move itself by having a clear sense of how you will go about meeting new friends or spending your days. If possible, make several visits to your new community before you move permanently. If you want to buy a home or an apartment, try to rent first.

Give yourself six months to a year to settle in. Expect to feel out of sorts (or unhappy) the first few months after moving. Before concluding that your decision was a mistake, understand that any major change is stressful. No matter how much people plan ahead, it takes time to settle in mentally. Finding yourself may be around the corner, even when the chance of ever being happy seems remote.

Moving to Florida was my wife's idea. Raised in Europe, I tolerated an adulthood spent in New York City but felt out of

Table 5   Checklist for Evaluating a Continuing Care Community

Paying for Services

1. Check with several communities in the general area that offer similar services and contracts to determine if your community's fees are competitive.
2. Find out how you are expected to pay for services and under what conditions your monthly charges will be raised or lowered.
3. Know the policy for residents who become unable to pay the monthly charges.
4. Receive assurance in writing that any large payment you are making to reserve a place in the community will be returned if you decide not to enter.
5. Make sure the contract spells out the terms for refunding your fees if you terminate your contract. How much money will be refunded if you leave voluntarily or involuntarily? What will happen to your investment if you die?
6. Find out how long your living unit will be maintained (and what adjustment will be made in your monthly fee) if you are transferred to another place such as a nursing home.
7. Find out in what circumstances your contract can be terminated and under what conditions you can be transferred within or out of the community. (For instance, what happens if the community decides you need the nursing home, but you do not want to go there?)

Sponsorship and Management

1. Learn who sponsors or owns the community, and have their financial and other relationships to the community spelled out.
2. Find out who is on the board of directors and what their responsibilities to the community are.
3. Meet the administrator and try to evaluate his or her competence.
4. Review a copy of the rules and regulations. Find out what input residents have in establishing the rules. (Be wary of highly restrictive regulations or of very few rules.)
5. Discuss the community with the staff and, most important, its residents. How do they feel about the way the community is being run? What are the pros and cons of being a resident?
6. Find out if the community is properly certified.
7. Ask about admissions policies and requirements.

Table 5   (Continued)

The Financial Condition
1. Discuss the community's annual report and other relevant documents with a financial adviser.
2. Get a copy of the community's most recent audit and determine what reserves it holds.

Shelter, Services, and Care
1. Find out exactly what is covered by your fees and what is extra.
2. Determine how often and for how long each service is provided, and be sure these facts are clearly stated in your contract.
3. Tour the nursing home or health-care facility and meet with the medical director and staff. Sample the other services (such as meals) and ask the residents how they feel about the quality of what is being offered.

Signing the Contract
1. Review the contract with your lawyer.
2. Review the contract with the community administrator or other person in authority.

Note: Use relevant questions to evaluate any retirement community.

sorts moving south for what I thought would be a mindless retirement life. My prejudices were wrong. I found a job teaching at the local university—something I could never do in Europe or New York without a Ph.D. I am respected and known here in this smaller pond. And once I scratched the surface, those shallow-seeming Floridians proved to be interesting companions after all. But for almost the whole first year, I was planning my escape. I'm so glad I held on long enough to find out I really do like it here.

If you are unhappy with your current home and have the choice, it makes sense to lean toward moving, even if you are not sure things will work out. Taking a chance that has the potential to make life much better seems a fair risk. Even misplaced moves are not irrevocable. They are just easier or harder to undo, depending on how carefully you build in an escape hatch. So go, but with the idea that if a year has passed and you are still unhappy, you will think seriously about returning. Of the nine thousand older people who moved from Florida to New York in 1984, many were probably migrating back from their retirement homes. Granted, some may have been forced to return because of poor health; but others surely moved back voluntarily. They simply realized their original decision was wrong.

New Options for Homeowners

If you are like most people, you prefer not to move. You may own your house, and selling may be unthinkable. But the liabilities of being a homeowner may mean staying is not ideal either. To help you, some interesting innovations have been devised.[21]

If you are a homeowner and your income is limited, the pressure to sell the house and live better on the proceeds can be great. In the past you had to select from two unhappy alternatives: "Stay where I want to be and be economically strapped, or move where I don't want to go to get the extra cash." With what are called home-equity conversion plans, you can have more money and still remain in your home.

HOME-EQUITY PLANS

These plans are essentially variations of three familiar transactions: loans, sales, and deferred payments.

In *home-equity loan plans*, you arrange for a reverse mortgage (or what is called an adjustable-rate reverse mortgage or reverse shared-appreciation mortgage), exchanging equity for cash while retaining title to your property and continuing to occupy your home. Each month the lender, usually a bank or a savings and loan association, sends you a check. These checks are a loan that must eventually be repaid with interest. But you do not have to pay the money back until a specified period has elapsed—five or ten years or until you sell the home or die. In most cases your home is ultimately sold to repay the debt, though you can use a short-term reverse mortgage to pay living expenses until a pension or other source of income comes in. When your home is sold, any value beyond the debt goes to you or your estate.

Home-equity sale plans differ in that you lose title to your home. In one type, for instance, called a sale-leaseback plan, you sell your home to an investor who immediately leases it back to you for life. You become a renter in the home you have just sold.

The February 1987 issue of the *Gerontologist* described a Marin County home-equity demonstration project, recently expanded to San Francisco and eight other California counties (Alameda, San Mateo, Santa Clara, Contra Costa, Sonoma, Sacramento, Napa, and Orange).[22] The program offers eligible applicants financial counseling and a choice of either a home-equity loan plan or a sale-leaseback plan. Most people who participate choose the loan plan to help pay for long-term home health care.

Home equity is not widely available. For instance, to be eligible for this California program, applicants must be sixty-two or over, have a low or moderate income and modest assets, own their homes outright, and live in one of the counties the project serves. Because programs are expensive to run, home equity may never be widespread, though the idea is catching on. There are now demonstration projects in Tucson, Boston, Milwaukee, and Nassau County, New York. There is even one in Musashino, Japan. From the National Center on Home Equity in Madison, Wisconsin (see the end of this chapter), you can find out whether such a program exists in your community.

If you are "house rich" but not eligible for home-equity plans, you have other options. For example, suppose money is not a major concern, but the size of your house is. You feel uncomfortable living alone in a four-bedroom home, rattling around where a family would fit. Your house is unwieldy, hard to clean, heat, and maintain. You hate finding someone to mow the lawn. You are frightened of being by yourself. What would happen in a robbery or a medical emergency? Still, you refuse to sell.

ACCESSORY APARTMENTS

One solution may be to install an accessory apartment in your home and rent it out.[23] An accessory apartment is a second, private living unit in the extra space of a single-family home.

The cost of installing such an apartment can be relatively low, depending on the design of your house.

Renting out an accessory apartment will offer you the security of having someone living nearby. It also may be possible to arrange for your tenant to do some services around the house in return for a reduction in rent. And the additional income will be a bonus even if you are not short of cash.

Before considering this architectural modification, check with your local zoning agency. In some areas accessory apartments are illegal. In some age is a condition for approval: you or the person living in your unit must be sixty-two or over. Some communities allow conversion only for relatives.

Options for
Low-Income Nonhomeowners

If you do not own a home and your income is tight, you might consider a solution that has always been popular with single people starting out—sharing the cost with someone else.[24]

HOUSING MATCH-UP SERVICES

A growing number of services make finding a compatible housemate easier by linking people with others they are likely to live comfortably with. Some of these housing match-up services are for older people only, but some are intergenerational; you may be matched with a person of any age. To find out whether a service of this type is available in your community, write or call the Shared Housing Resource Center in Philadelphia (see the end of this chapter.)

Leah Dobkin, director of this national clearinghouse, advises selecting a housing match-up service that offers counseling—one where a trained person explores your expectations, doubts, and concerns about having a housemate. Counseling is important to help people sort out whether they really are prepared to enter an arrangement of this type.

Or go it on your own. If you are a homeowner, advertise in your local newspaper for a boarder; or offer your services as a baby-sitter in exchange for a room in a single-family house.

(Once again, check your local zoning laws to see if renting out a single-family house is legal.)

Many people shy away from having a housemate out of fear: "What if things don't work out?" Though a bad experience is always a possibility, taking these precautions will lessen your risk.

1. Carefully spell out the details of your arrangement in writing (chores, who pays for what, etc.) before the move.

2. Spend some time with a potential housemate. Would it be possible to give living together a month's trial? Could you go away together for a weekend to get to know one another? At least conduct a thorough interview. As Dobkin advises, "The time to negotiate a workable arrangement is before you commit yourself to it, economically, physically, emotionally."

SUBSIDIZED HOUSING AND RENTAL ASSISTANCE

Another choice you may have is subsidized housing.[25] The government provides financial assistance to churches and synagogues, civic organizations, private developers, and consumer cooperatives who then build and manage housing for people with incomes below a certain amount. Some low-income housing for the elderly is of better quality than retirement housing at almost any price. Innovative architectural design, carefully planned access to community services, effective management, and a rich blend of on-site options makes some subsidized housing developments national showcases of good planning and design.

Subsidized housing ranges from apartments for people with no physical impairments to units providing meals, housekeeping, and social services to older people in frail health. And while most programs do require that people earn less than a certain amount to qualify, some do not.

Unfortunately, because of its desirability, the best subsidized housing tends to have a long waiting list. By asking your local office for the aging, your local housing authority, or HUD (the United States Department of Housing and Urban Development), you can find out what is available in your area. Information about one program, sponsored by the Farmers Home Administration (FmHA) of the United States Department of Agriculture, can be gotten from the FmHA office in your area. Your area HUD and FmHA offices also will have information about another program you may qualify for—government assistance with your rent if your income is below a certain amount.

Sponsored by HUD and FmHA Rental assistance operates in a similar way. With a certificate of eligibility from the agency, you search for rental housing, either in your current building, in another apartment, or in a private or federally assisted apartment complex. You pay a maximum of 30 percent of your income for rent, and the government pays the rest based on a "fair market rent" they approve. If you qualify for this type of assistance, you also may get help with large housing expenses such as utility charges. However—as with subsidized housing—the funds for this type of assistance are inadequate to cover the number of eligible applicants.

No matter·what your financial situation, investigate your choices if you are at all dissatisfied with where you live now. Go beyond this chapter, which has focused mainly on alternatives for older adults. Explore every option without fear. The research shows that if you plan wisely, you need not be afraid of the mental or physical consequences of making a change.

For More Information

GENERAL RESOURCES

Carlin, V. E., and R. Mansberg. *Where Can Mom Live? A Family Guide to Living Arrangements for Elderly Parents.* Lexington, Mass., Lexington Books, 1987.

Covers much of the information in this chapter in more depth—housing alternatives, modifying one's home, guidelines on how to plan a move.

Crosby, R., and T. Flynn, eds. *Housing for Older Adults: Options and Answers.* Washington, D.C.: National Council on the Aging, 1986.

An overview of housing for older Americans. Nationally recognized experts discuss current and future housing needs and programs.

Dickinson, P. A. *Sunbelt Retirement.* Mount Prospect, Ill.: AARP Books, 1986.

Offers practical information and advice on retiring to the Sunbelt. Each of the thirteen Sunbelt states is discussed individually. A rating scale evaluates the major retirement areas in each state.

Hubbard, L., and T. Beck, eds. *Housing Options for Older Americans.* Washington, D.C.: AARP, 1984.

Discusses the housing options available to older people as well as providing information on how to modify your home.

Sumichrast, M., R. G. Safer, and M. Sumichrast. *Planning Your Retirement Housing.* Mount Prospect, Ill.: AARP Books, 1984.

Discusses issues such as housing costs, design, whether to move or not. Outlines strategies for preparing for retirement.

RETIREMENT COMMUNITIES

American Association of Homes for the Aging. *The Continuing Care Retirement Community: A Guidebook for Consumers.* Washington, D.C.: American Association of Homes for the Aging, 1984.

Offers information on what issues to consider and how to evaluate continuing-care contracts.

National Directory of Retirement Facilities. Phoenix: Oryx Press, 1985.

Lists over twelve thousand retirement facilities, their type, and who to make contact with by state and city.

Rapier, A. T., ed. *National Continuing Care Directory.* Mount Prospect, Ill.: AARP Books, 1984.

Provides data about each of the four hundred continuing-care communities that existed as of 1984.

ACCESSORY APARTMENTS

Hare, P. C., S. Dwight, and M. Dwight. *Accessory Apartments: Using Surplus Space in Single Family Houses.* Chicago: American Planning Association, 1981.

Addresses the issues to consider in installing accessory apartments.

HOME MATCHING AND SHARED HOUSING

Bierbrier, D. *Living with Tenants.* Arlington, Va.: Housing Connection, 1982.

Practical guide on how to rent a house to tenants, find and keep
responsible people, charge a fair rent, and so forth.

Horne, J. *Home Sharing: New Lifestyles for People over Fifty.* Washington, D.C.: AARP Books, 1987.
Discusses legal issues and decisions related to shared housing.

Shared Housing Resource Center, 6344 Greene Street, Philadelphia, Pennsylvania 19144   (215) 848-1220.
National organization promoting shared housing for older people
locally, regionally, and nationally. Also publishes materials.

HOME EQUITY

National Center for Home Equity Conversion, 110 East Main, Room
605, Madison, Wisconsin 53703   (608) 256-2111.
National center for information on home-equity issues. Also publishes materials.

PART

IV

DISEASE

CHAPTER

9

DEMENTIA

The person whose mind I have always envied most, my brilliant childhood friend who became a historian, has Alzheimer's disease. Several years ago she began noticing changes in her teaching. She had trouble finding the right word for what she wanted to say. Sometimes she would pause in the middle of a sentence and begin a thought again. We all thought her complaints were psychological. She was too upset about her daughter's divorce. We understood there was something seriously wrong only on our trip to Europe in the summer of 1984.

Janet had to ask the tour guide for the schedule several times a day. She could not keep the time the bus would leave in her head. She would ask questions about sights that had been discussed only a few minutes before. She seemed apathetic, not thrilled, when we visited the historical places I knew she loved. Restaurants were a problem. She had trouble finding her way back to our table after trips to the ladies' room. Once we caught her about to walk out the door. Afterward I made excuses so I could take her there and back.

Over the next year or so she was able to handle life fairly well once back in the familiar surroundings of our town. She took a sabbatical from teaching but went to her office to "work" on papers several days a week. Everyone felt it would be good for her keep up the pretense, even though she could no longer really produce. Jack let her to do everything—shop, cook, take care of the house. He never stopped her from going out alone. But he was always upset. Would this be the time she took the car and wound up lost or dead? Would this dinner be the one where the stove was left on? By then she had been seen by specialists. Everyone knew what she probably had.

This year things have gotten much worse. My cool, rational friend now has outbursts of anger that come from left field. She sometimes is unable to sit still for more than a second at a time. When she is home she wants to go out. Once out, she wants to go back. She is like a person possessed—a firecracker of emotions without purpose or will.

Last week I invited Jack and her to dinner. When I would go into the kitchen, Janet would get up to go to the door. Jack would have to jump up, bring her back, and explain we were about to eat, only to have her pop up again. When I finally got dinner on the table, he had to cut her food and serve her. I was near tears by the time they left. What's going on? Can't anything be done to ease her suffering? What about me? What is my chance of getting this terrible disease?

Senility is everyone's worst terror about old age. The flood of publicity about Alzheimer's disease has multiplied this concern. We hear there is an epidemic; there is nothing medical science can do. But we know little else about this sword hanging over our later years: "Is my forgetting names more often a sign of beginning Alzheimer's disease?" "Is becoming senile the inevitable price if we live to a ripe old age?" *"What is senility?"*

Senility Is Dementia

The medical term for senility is dementia. Dementia refers to a set of symptoms, not a single illness—a generally progressive, irreversible decline in memory, reasoning, thinking. A number of diseases produce this inexorable intellectual deterioration. Though it has now become the popular catchword for everything, Alzheimer's disease is only the most common of them.

THE SYMPTOMS

When people have dementia (caused either by Alzheimer's disease or by another illness) an early sign is trouble in remembering the ongoing events of daily life. A woman may forget she just made a phone call and call her daughter back. She may not remember driving to the store an hour earlier and may make a second trip.

Sometimes the first symptom is a change in personality. The person withdraws, becoming apathetic, abstracted. Or a life that had been tightly ordered seems to unravel. A fastidious housekeeper begins leaving the dinner dishes in the sink; her immaculate house is now in disarray. A dapper, punctual man regularly shows up at work hours late, disheveled, with a stained tie.

Changes like these are almost always either isolated incidents (How many of us have never blanked out on a phone call we made two seconds ago?) or signs that something is wrong with the emotional side of life. Personal problems may be preoccupying us, affecting our memory, our mood, our ability to handle life competently. *It is very difficult to be sure a person is suffering from a dementing illness when the condition is in its earliest stages.*

Strange or unusual behavior is often seen in retrospect as the first sign of the disease when, as the months pass, the victim's mental processes deteriorate. For instance, when University of Michigan researchers interviewed family members of dementia victims, many said they had interpreted early symptoms in their loved ones, later diagnosed as Alzheimer's disease, as emotional problems.[1] When their mother became forgetful, children decided she was depressed or deliberately tuning them out. When a husband started behaving strangely, his wife might worry about their marriage. Some women even went for counseling or considered divorce.

Even if a family sensed what was really happening early on, they were often unable to articulate exactly what was peculiar or amiss and so had trouble convincing the doctor to take their worries seriously. Months might go by before the true condition was diagnosed.

If the problem is a dementing illness, things do get worse; eventually it becomes obvious that something is very wrong. As the illness reaches its middle stages, a person's reasoning becomes strangely concrete. A man may be unable to follow simple instructions such as "turn right to Main Street" or "twist the cap to open the jar." The advice to "just dive in" may be greeted by the puzzled comment, "I'm not near a swimming pool!"

Simple calculations become difficult. A woman may first have trouble making change, then forget that four quarters make a dollar, then not understand the word dollar. She may be unable to name objects correctly or remember their function—calling forks spoons, spearing steak with her knife, cutting food with her spoon. Judgment becomes increasingly unreliable, alarming family members. Children, worried at first that Mom might cross Main Street against a red light and be hit by a car, months later may find that their anxiety multiplies: "Will she run out on Main Street undressed?"

In the final stages there is profound disorientation, an inability to locate oneself in time or space. People are often unable to dress or feed themselves, control their bowels, remember their names, or recognize their families.

Barry Gurland, director of geriatric psychiatry at Columbia University and an expert on dementia's clinical course, thinks the intellectual losses that occur as this dreadful condition advances are like peeling an onion.[2] As time goes by, each cognitive milestone is stripped away in the reverse of the order in which it was attained. So first a person loses the mental skills acquired in adolescence—complicated abstract thought—then what was learned in elementary school—reading, the ability to add and subtract. Finally, the milestones reached at ages two and one are gone—dressing, forming sentences, going to the toilet.

Another expert on dementia's clinical course, Penn State psychologist Steve Zarit, believes this analogy is misleading.[3] In his experience, not everyone changes in this lockstep way. Some people never become incontinent. Others, while unable to control their bladder or bowels, may retain even complex skills if they were passionate pursuits before the disease struck. A gourmet cook might still prepare meals even though she can no longer remember her husband's name. A concert pianist may continue to play even though he needs help getting dressed.

Zarit's research shows that the disease often has an emotional course too. In the middle stages of the illness, very difficult behavior such as aimless wandering, or night waking, or intense hostility toward loved ones tends to erupt. As more abilities are lost, people tend to quiet down. Ironically, in interviewing spouses caring for Alzheimer's patients, Zarit and his colleagues found that as the illness reached its final stages, caregivers paradoxically found it easier to cope, largely because when the deterioration became profound the disruptive behavior abated.[4]

Not everyone develops these difficult symptoms when the disease is in its middle stages. For instance, in tracking people with Alzheimer's disease, University of Washington researchers found that only about 10 to 15 percent of their subjects ever became severely agitated or abusive.[5] When people do lash out at loved ones—accusing a husband or wife of poisoning them, disowning a caring daughter or son—the reason is physical, not personal. The disease is destroying areas of the brain involved in modulating the emotions. It is not laying bare the true self or real feelings. *Our real self is the one we have when our faculties are intact.*

Perhaps the most heartbreaking aspect of this illness, however, is that we cannot predict how rapidly it will progress. Some people get worse very quickly, becoming unable to understand the basics of life within a few months after they are diagnosed; others may stay at about the same mental level for years. On average, people live a few years from the time they are diagnosed. But some die within six months and, with excellent care, others can live twenty years.[6] So planning for the future becomes difficult, as a family either prays that the loved one will not get worse or yearns for the death that will end the pain.

Though dementia is a leading cause of death, the brain impairment itself is not what directly kills. In fact, at the 1986 annual meeting of the Gerontological Society of America, doctors from the Jewish Institute for Geriatric Care in New York reported that the Alzheimer's patients were healthier than the average older person their health center served.[7] As the illness progresses, physical problems related to the mental losses arise that do cause death. A man may forget to swallow and

choke on a piece of food; a woman may develop pneumonia
from months of being in bed.

CAUSES

Although there are a handful of rare dementing illnesses, two
distinct diseases are typically responsible for the dementia
people develop in later life: Alzheimer's disease and multi-infarct dementia. Because it is the top-ranked cause of old-age
dementia, Alzheimer's disease has been in the spotlight; however, only a bare majority (about 50 to 60 percent) of the older
people who have dementia have Alzheimer's disease alone;
about 15 percent have dementia of the multi-infarct type; in
25 percent of cases mental impairment is caused by the ravages of the two diseases combined.[8]

Though the way they affect memory and thinking looks
similar or even identical, multi-infarct dementia and Alzheimer's disease damage the brain very differently. Multi-infarct dementia attacks the vascular system—the blood vessels
nourishing the brain; Alzheimer's disease is an illness of the
neurons (brain cells) themselves.

Multi-Infarct Dementia

"Hardening of the arteries" is the way people have described
the vascular (blood vessel) problem called multi-infarct dementia. In the past, this colloquial description was a good one,
because experts thought that "hardened" and partially
clogged arteries produced this particular form of dementia.
Today we know that this vascular type of dementia is caused
not by partially blocked arteries, but by completely blocked
ones. A series of small strokes (or in medical terminology,
multi-infarcts) is what produces the changes in memory and
thinking.

A stroke occurs when a blood vessel feeding the brain becomes blocked, the blood supply is cut off, and the part of the
brain nourished by that vessel either is damaged or dies. A
large stroke produces symptoms that are impossible to miss—
paralysis, loss of speech, perhaps death. With multi-infarct de-

mentia, strokes are so minor that individually they may cause only transient symptoms or no distinct symptoms at all. But as their number increases and more and more brain tissue dies, intellectual processes gradually get worse.

If you have had a large stroke you are not predestined to suffer from multi-infarct dementia, though you may run a greater risk of developing this disease. Many people who have a large stroke never have multi-infarct dementia, and many people who suffer from multi-infarct dementia never have a large stroke.[9]

The best treatment for multi-infarct dementia is prevention—reducing the risk factors for any type of stroke: control your blood pressure, your weight, your cholesterol; stop smoking.[10] Although there is no way of reversing damage that has already been done, making these changes may help slow the illness's downward course. Unfortunately, there is no way of preventing or slowing the ravages of that most feared enemy of old age—Alzheimer's disease.

Alzheimer's Disease

Alzheimer's disease attacks our humanity at its core, destroying the brain cells themselves. A healthy, normal neuron looks like a tree. In Alzheimer's disease it is as if the tree is slowly being killed by a blight. First it loses its branches, then it swells and becomes gnarled. Finally, its trunk decays and it becomes a stump.[11] Abnormal structures replace normal cells: long, wavy filaments called neurofibrillary tangles and thick bits of protein called senile plaques.

The neural devastation advances much like the gypsy moth plague that spread from forest to forest about ten years ago, eventually covering much of the Northeast. At the beginning there are just a few changes in limited areas of the brain. One section that tends to be heavily affected early on is the hippocampus—the part of the brain responsible for solidifying (or encoding) new memories—explaining why one of the first symptoms of Alzheimer's disease is difficulty in remembering recent events. Gradually the damage cuts a wider swath. The cortex (our brain's reasoning center) is studded with abnormal brain fragments; if the disease is advanced, in some places there may be few normal neurons left.

WHAT ARE THE CAUSES?

Many researchers speculate that rather than having a single cause, Alzheimer's disease may be the outcome of several types of insults to the brain. While we do not know exactly what causes this mysterious illness, theories have centered on these agents of destruction.[12]

A virus. Because a virus is known to produce a very rare type of dementia, some researchers think—even though none has been found—that a slow-acting virus, one taking years to incubate in the body, might be implicated in Alzheimer's disease. *But there is no evidence of anyone's ever catching Alzheimer's disease from someone else.*

A disorder of the immune system. Another hypothesis is that an immune system "error" may be partly to blame. In 1987 researchers at Rockefeller University reported finding abnormal antibodies in patients with Alzheimer's disease;[13] they speculate that these antibodies, instead of functioning normally to destroy outside invaders such as viruses, may attack the blood/brain barrier, the vital chemical sheath that keeps injurious substances from gaining access to the brain. Once the integrity of the blood/brain barrier is breached, a virus or other harmful substance might gain access to the brain and set off the disease.

Aluminum. Besides a virus, a strong candidate for instigating Alzheimer's disease is aluminum, because a striking feature of the brains of Alzheimer's victims is an abnormal concentration of this particular element. Does absorbing too much aluminum over a lifetime play any part in producing the disease? So far, laboratory studies of this hypothesis have been negative; but because high aluminum levels are such an important feature of the illness, many scientists think this substance is likely to play some role in the puzzle of Alzheimer's disease.

A genetic defect. Without doubt, the most exciting new research lead involves genetics. In 1987 scientists at Massachusetts General Hospital reported identifying a genetic defect in people with a strong family history of Alzheimer's disease.[14]

The Alzheimer's-related genetic marker is found on chromosome number 21, the very chromosome that is duplicated in people suffering from the birth defect Down's syndrome. For several years researchers had been tantalized by what they knew was an important connection between these two illnesses, because victims of Down's syndrome (mongolism) universally develop Alzheimer's disease if they live to age forty. Now the mystery is solved. Having an extra chromosome 21 may be giving people victimized by Down's syndrome the Alzheimer's-related genetic program in spades.

Other research reported in the February 1987 issue of *Science* suggests that the illness may be set off by abnormal deposits of a protein called amyloid accumulating in the brain.[15] Amyloid is a major component of senile plaques and neurofibrillary tangles—the abnormal structures that replace the normal neurons. Do the genetic instructions "produce amyloid" trigger Alzheimer's disease directly by causing this toxic protein to build up? Does an Alzheimer's gene (or set of genes) act in concert with a chemical such as aluminum or with a virus to produce these harmful deposits? Whatever the answer, some scientists now believe amyloid is central to the mystery of this devastating disease.

WHAT IS YOUR RISK OF GETTING ALZHEIMER'S DISEASE?

Finding a genetic marker for Alzheimer's disease brings us a step closer to developing a test to tell what a person's chances are of getting this terrible disease. However, because scientists are just beginning to unravel the genetic determinants of the illness, this test may be years away. Statistics must suffice to answer that anxious question, "How likely am I to get Alzheimer's disease?"

If you have a strong family history—if several close family members developed the disease unusually early, before sixty or so—you do run a real risk. Otherwise the statistics are very comforting. Your chance of developing Alzheimer's disease (or any other form of dementia) is small, at least until advanced old age. Alzheimer's disease (and other old-age dementias) are illnesses of very late life—extremely rare before age sixty, uncommon but rising gradually in prevalence over the next two decades. As table 6 shows, real vulnerability begins in the mid-eighties, when a significant minority of people do have serious memory problems. However, even among people hardy enough in body to live to one hundred, many survive sound in mind.

Interpret these statistics cautiously; the proportion of people with memory problems at each age varies greatly depending on the study we pick. The reason is not necessarily that older people in Japan are less (or more) prone to senility than residents of New York State but that the criteria for judging problems differ from survey to survey. And even some people diagnosed as having severe memory problems do not have dementia. They may have a treatable condition or even no intellectual deficit at all.

Getting an Accurate Diagnosis

Because no technological advance has enabled us to see into the brain to prove that Alzheimer's disease (or multi-infarct dementia) is there, experts estimate that an alarming 20 to 30 percent of the time people are wrongly diagnosed as having dementia when they actually have a treatable disease.[16] Doctors may leap to a diagnosis of dementia in an older patient because they are conditioned to think that old age equals senility and are not skilled enough (or willing) to do the fine-grained testing needed to judge whether a dementing illness really does exist. The diagnosis of Alzheimer's disease is made by exclusion, after a full medical and psychological evaluation has been done (see below) and when every other explanation for mental changes has been ruled out. Proof can be obtained only by autopsy, when the brain is examined directly. A surprising number of reversible conditions can look like Alzheimer's disease.

Depression. On the surface, depression seems to have nothing in common with dementia. How can an emotional disorder look like pathology of the intellect? The reason is that a cardinal symptom of depression is intellectual change—cloudy thinking, problems in focusing, trouble in remembering what is going on. Unfortunately, these intellectual

Table 6 Percentage of People with Dementia at Different Ages in
Selected Community Surveys

Survey	Age				
	65–69	70–74	75–79	80–84	85+
Japan (N = 531)	1.9	2.7	11.3	9.9	33.3
Denmark (N = 978)	2.1	4.0	7.8	12.6	21.4
Syracuse, New York (N = 1,805)	3.7	5.4	9.3	8.8	23.7
England (N = 758)	2.4	2.9	5.6	22.0[a]	
Sweden (N = 443)	0.9	5.1[b]		21.8[a]	

Source: Adapted from D. W. Kay and K. Bergmann, "The Epidemiology of Mental Disorder among the Aged in the Community," in *Handbook of Mental Health and Aging,* ed. J. Birren and R. B. Sloane (Englewood Cliffs, N.J.: Prentice-Hall, 1980).
Note: Dementia is defined as moderate or severe problems with memory or thinking.
[a]Aged eighty and over.
[b]Aged seventy to seventy-nine.

changes often appear in depressed older people without the gloomy attitude that cues doctors to depression—making the two illnesses sometimes very difficult to distinguish.

Physical illnesses. Because being sick almost always clouds our thinking, practically any illness can potentially be mistaken for dementia—the flu, an earache, even a bad cold. However, these illnesses in particular can produce the chronic mental confusion that makes a false diagnosis a special risk: metabolic problems such as thyroid dysfunction, kidney failure, Addison's disease, hypoglycemia; cancer of the lung, breast, or other tissues; neurological disorders such as brain tumors, parkinsonism, meningitis; and kidney and bladder infections.[17]

Memory problems mislabeled dementia may occur after surgery, following an accident, or even from lying in bed for a few weeks. A person who is profoundly deaf may appear demented. If you ask your ninety-year-old mother a question and she stares blankly at you, it is surprisingly hard to tell whether the problem is her ears or her mind. A heart attack can be misdiagnosed as dementia too. Among the elderly, about 13 percent of the time mental confusion is its main or only symptom.

Medications. Medicines can impair thinking in people of any age. But drug-induced mental confusion is much more likely in later life, because our body metabolizes medications less effectively and we are more likely to be taking several types of drugs regularly.

People who take L-dopa, steroids, gentamicin, digitalis, antihypertensive medications, or tranquilizers are at special risk of being misdiagnosed as demented, because high doses of these drugs in particular produce symptoms that can look very much like Alzheimer's disease. A poignant 1985 study involving the tranquilizer Valium amply demonstrates this. When researchers gave normal older people ten milligrams of Valium—a dose that, while large, is within the range a doctor might prescribe—they had problems on a memory test that were very similar to those of a comparison group suffering from Alzheimer's disease.[18]

We all accepted that Mom was getting senile. She forgot things, seemed confused about where she was much of the time, and would often break off to stare into space. Then in the hospital they took her off all the pills she had been taking, and it was as if twenty years were erased from her age. From a zombie she returned to the world of the living. Her mind was as sharp as it had been at fifty!

Delirium is the medical term for the mental confusion many drugs and diseases cause. A person who rapidly becomes very confused and disoriented—within a few hours or days—is usually suffering from delirium.[19] The hallmark of dementia is slow progression. Although people with dementia do vary in how well they can think on different days, when someone becomes delirious the shifts are dramatic—a rational human being is there one hour, the next a madman appears. And the delirious person may really look mad—perhaps seeing things on the wall or babbling incoherently. If you witness this type of transformation, get medical help *immediately*. The person may have a life-threatening problem or one that can cause permanent brain damage if not treated right away.

WHERE TO GO AND WHAT TESTS TO EXPECT

Because diagnosing dementia can be so tricky, if you suspect a relative may have Alzheimer's disease, bypass your family doctor. Visit someone with special training—an internist, a neurologist, a psychiatrist, or a psychologist who is trained in geriatrics. Preferably, get your relative evaluated at a hospital-based geriatric center.

Visiting a center is preferable to seeing any sole practitioner for several reasons: experts from several disciplines will collaborate in making the diagnosis; procedures and diagnostic tests are more likely to be state of the art; the fee may be less prohibitive (Medicare will pay for most of the cost in any case, because dementia has been reclassified from a psychiatric to a neurological disorder); and if your fears are justified and the problem is dementia, you will be thoroughly briefed on your options and on what to expect.

We would imagine that any humane doctor would sit down with a family and carefully explain the situation after delivering a diagnosis of this magnitude. Not true! In the University of Michigan study of family members discussed earlier in this chapter, most people gave shocking accounts of how they were told the facts.[20] Some said that the curt words, "He will gradually deteriorate, becoming completely helpless," were delivered in a waiting room or an elevator. Or the same diagnosis might be heedlessly offered while the patient was standing right there. Not only were families understandably bitter about this insensitivity, they were left ill equipped to understand the problems they would eventually have. Of the 289 people in this study, only three said their doctors had called a family conference to thoroughly explain what the diagnosis meant.

My mother had been getting confused at night, so we took her to a highly recommended neurologist. He saw her for literally five minutes and me for another five, then pronounced her senile and told me to start looking for a nursing home. There was no physical examination, no understanding that I might not want to put her away. Later, by accident, I found out from a friend how many choices I really had!

For a referral to a center where you will get a top-quality assessment and counseling, call your local office of the aging or local chapter of the Alzheimer's Disease and Related Disorders Association (this helpful organization also operates a twenty-four-hour toll-free information hotline: [800] 621-0379). The National Institute on Aging, which coordinates research on Alzheimer's disease, has designated these ten hospitals, associated with medical schools, as centers for the diagnosis, treatment, and dissemination of information about dementia: Duke University; Harvard Medical School/Massachusetts General Hospital; Johns Hopkins University; Mount Sinai School of Medicine/Bronx Veterans Administration Medical Center; University of California, San Diego; University of Kentucky; University of Pittsburgh; University of Southern California; University of Washington; and Washington University, Saint Louis.

If you visit one of these centers or another (top-quality dementia services are now available in almost every metropolitan area), expect the following diagnostic procedures and tests.[21]

A history of the problem. Because a pattern of insidious development is a major clue indicating dementia, a primary diagnostic tool is a careful medical history. When you visit, be prepared to describe exactly what has been going on. How long have you noticed the problems? Have the symptoms gotten progressively worse? What difficulties were there to begin with, and what occur now? Did any event—an illness, a loss such as widowhood, or a fall—predate the problems?

You will be asked about current and past illnesses, depression, the medications your relative is taking. Because chemical toxins can cause memory problems, you may be asked about long-term exposure to chemicals.

A complete physical and neurological examination. A thorough physical examination will be done. Urine will be tested; blood will be drawn; neurological and memory tests may be administered. Particularly if the impairments are subtle, a psychologist may administer a battery of neuropsychological tests. These tests, which can be invaluable in the differential diagnosis of dementia, are somewhat like the paper-and-pencil measures of abilities we get in school.

Measures of brain function. An EEG, a CAT scan, or a PET scan may also be given. The EEG (electroencephalogram) measures the electrical activity of different areas of the brain. Electrodes are attached to the scalp, and a machine traces brain waves.

The CAT scan and PET scan, also safe, painless procedures, provide pictures of the brain. The CAT scan is like an X-ray in three dimensions. A computer generates a picture of the brain's mass. The PET scan measures the brain's consumption of glucose. By using this newer, only occasionally available test, doctors can tell which areas of the brain are functioning well (metabolizing glucose normally) and which are not (areas where glucose consumption is abnormally low).

The CAT scan can rule out other reasons for mental changes such as brain tumors. When the PET scan shows extensive areas of low glucose metabolism, it can confirm that dementia is severe; but neither test can prove the existence of a condition such as Alzheimer's disease. Although both techniques are wonderful for diagnosing other neurological conditions, neither allows the direct examination of the brain cells that is necessary to positively diagnose Alzheimer's disease.

Luckily, despite the difficulty of absolutely proving a person has dementia, if you do visit a center staffed by knowledgeable professionals, you can have confidence in the diagnosis you get. When researchers followed two hundred patients evaluated at a geriatric clinic specializing in the diagnosis and treatment of dementia for a year, they found very few diagnostic mistakes. If a person had been diagnosed as having dementia, over time that diagnosis was almost always confirmed.[22]

Treatment

Although there is no way to prevent or medically treat Alzheimer's disease, experimental drugs and procedures are feverishly being tried. If an experimental treatment is available to your relative, check the reputability of the procedure and the qualifications of the researchers doing the study with the National Institute on Aging. As I mentioned earlier, the NIA coordinates research on Alzheimer's disease. Then ask the researchers doing the study to carefully describe any risks of the treatment. While you might think (with some reason) that anything is worth a try, consider the possibility that the treatment might have a side effect that either is life threatening or makes things worse. Hopeless diagnoses such as Alzheimer's disease render people vulnerable to dangerous or expensive quack remedies. So be on special guard against being victimized.

If your relative is enrolled in a legitimate experimental study, be careful not to get your hopes up too far. At most the substances being tested purport to slow up the inexorable course of Alzheimer's disease or improve the patient's capacities a bit. No one claims to be able to restore everything that has been lost.

Several classes of drugs are now being tested on humans. The most intensively explored are medications that have the potential to stimulate the brain's production of the neurotransmitter acetylcholine. (The controversial drug THA, now undergoing clinical tests, is in this category.) For more than a decade scientists have known that a striking deficiency of this important neurotransmitter is characteristic of Alzheimer's disease.[23]

One reason progress in developing a memory-stimulating pill has been slow is that drugs that might be effective have trouble penetrating the blood/brain barrier, the sheath protecting the brain from anything foreign. Another roadblock is that a memory-enhancing drug has the best chance of being effective when the disease is in its beginning stages and the neural destruction is not too far advanced. However, it is precisely at this time that Alzheimer's disease can be so difficult to diagnose accurately.

The best way to keep informed about medical breakthroughs is to join the Alzheimer's Disease and Related Disorders Association, an excellent national organization begun and run by families of people with the disease. In addition to sponsoring research, serving as advocates for victims and their families, and setting up most of the support groups for caregiving families, the ADRDA publishes a newsletter that summarizes the most promising recent research. Becoming a member of this organization will also help you keep your feet on the ground. To be newsworthy, those tantalizing newspaper accounts of promising new leads sometimes tend to err on the "important breakthrough" side; the truth is we are *not* very close to finding a real cure for this tragic disease.

WHAT CAN BE DONE?

This does not mean that passivity and negativism are the best path. Taking the following steps may dramatically improve symptoms, capacities, and the quality of life.

Eliminate illnesses compounding the problem. Although it is incurable in itself, dementia often coexists with conditions that can be treated—depression, other illnesses, memory impairment from medications. These problems exacerbate the mental confusion. When they are ferreted out and eliminated, thinking often improves.[24]

Judiciously consider using tranquilizers. Although tranquilizers have the potential to make mental cloudiness worse, they can help with the emotional and behavioral symptoms of the disease. If a person with Alzheimer's disease wakes up at night to wander and scream, is physically abusive, is flooded with anxiety, or hears voices that are not there, antipsychotic medications, the same type of tranquilizer used to treat severe emotional disorders such as schizophrenia, may be worth a try. If your doctor does prescribe this type of medication, monitor your relative's symptoms carefully to see whether the net effect is genuinely better or worse.

Provide a simple, predictable environment. The environment also can have a marked effect on how well the person feels and functions. For instance, a man with Alzheimer's disease in its early stages may find work very threatening but have no trouble handling life comfortably if he retires and his mental requirements are less. Trips or moves are likely to be hard, because being in new territory puts extra stress on a mind struggling to make sense of a life already flowing by too fast. True, the pace is more relaxed in Arizona, but Chicago is where your wife has lived all her life. The neighborhood is too noisy, the house is too big; but the contours of each are imprinted on her brain. People with dementia function best on the most familiar ground.

My father used just the wrong approach with my mother during the years her memory was failing. He took her to every new restaurant, forced her to travel. He was trying to make her last years happy by offering her the best. He also believed that piling on more experiences was better—that it would strengthen the brain cells that remained. I wanted him to keep her life simple, not continually confront her with the terror of new things. It hurt me to see her humiliated, when she was forced to do things that were beyond her capacities, where all she could do was fail.

When a person's memory is dulled by an unstimulating life, new experiences may be the antidote. But dementia is totally different from the type of forgetting caused by looking at four walls. The advice to search out fulfillment or do memory exercises falls flat with dementia. No memory workout can retard the brain-cell loss of Alzheimer's disease. In fact, because it may flood the person with anxiety, forcing memory-stimulating exercises on an Alzheimer's victim is likely to boomerang.

Use external aids. On the other hand, using external memory props can be very effective, particularly when the illness is in its earlier stages. One standard prop is notes. Fasten a note to the stove reminding your mother to turn it off; pin one to the front door reminding your husband to take his coat. People with dementia tend to be more confused in the evening, in part because in the dark less information about the world comes in (and they also may be less alert). Simple strategies such as leaving a bathroom light on can reduce the terror of waking up with a full bladder and forgetting where the toilet is. In helping more information to penetrate, be creative! Use your ingenuity to turn up the volume of those things that must be remembered (see table 7).[25]

In the middle stages of the illness other devices may be very helpful—those that make living safer and assist the person with jobs such as bathing and dressing. If you are afraid your father will wander out of the house and get lost, install double locks, the kind that must be unlocked from the inside; sew identification labels in his clothing; there is even a homing device on the market that signals a caregiver when the patient wanders off.

Help for Caregivers

Keeping the environment predictable, buying helpful devices, and ruling out other memory-impairing conditions go only so far in reducing the strain of dealing with a person with this disease. The real effort lies in coping with a loved one turned alien, where the tools used in normal human encounters no longer apply.

Dave (who usually cared for his wife with dementia) had gone out of town the previous week and left his wife with their

Table 7　Devices to Aid Coping

Memory
Bulletin board for daily plans and messages
Kitchen timer and alarm watch as reminders

Safety
Sink overflow alarm (alarm sounds if water runs over)
Automatic shutoff kettle or teapot, iron, and stove
Childproof cabinet and door locks
Grab bars around toilet and bathtub
Appliance and light timers

Daily living
Clothes and shoes with Velcro closures (no buttons)
Gripping aids for toothbrushes, eating utensils, pens and pencils
Controlled-flow drinking cups
Doorknob extensions and handle restraints

Source: Adapted from J. O'Quinn, L. M. Street, S. Neal, and E. A. Wareham, *A Survey of Assistive Devices, Behavioral Management and Environmental Modifications for Use with the Cognitively Impaired Elderly* Oxford, Miss.: Living Systems, 1986. (The catalogs listed at the end of chap. 10 should have many of these products.)

daughter. After [they went] to a restaurant . . . Dave's wife
refused to get in the car to go back home. . . . She began accusing her daughter of trying to hurt her and insisted on seeing
Dave. They argued for some time but nothing calmed her down.
Instead, she got more and more agitated until she collapsed and
the paramedics were called. . . . When Dave arrived home, she
continued making accusations against their daughter. Dave
tried to reason with her but reported to the group that he had no
success. In fact, she denied having done anything wrong and insisted that it was her daughter's fault that she had gotten
upset.[26]

This incident, reported at a family support group session,
illustrates how emotionally difficult caring for someone with
dementia can be. It can take every ounce of forbearance to
cope full time with a person literally "out of his mind," as
many caregivers do.

For instance, in a 1986 study of caregivers, Duke University
researchers found that their subjects averaged three times as
many stress symptoms as a comparison group; they were
much more apt to use tranquilizers; they had low morale.
Hobbies, visits with their families and friends, and especially
just relaxing by themselves were all casualties to the burden of
dealing with this devastating disease. The one glimmer was
that physically these caregivers were holding up, no more
likely to visit their doctors than the control group—people
dealing with the normal stresses of daily life.[27]

It comes as no shock that caregiving causes emotional distress. The surprise is that the severity of the patient's illness
itself is not the primary determinant of that strain. Rather
than the victim's objective symptoms, three more external aspects of the situation seem to make caring for a person with
dementia feel impossibly burdensome: not having the support
of family and friends; having had an unloving or ambivalent
relationship with the person before the disease struck; and
feeling out of control, unable to handle problems that do
arise.[28]

Having a negative legacy from the past is hard to change.
But if you are caring for a victim of Alzheimer's disease you

can take action to draw on the other two resources that researchers find so critical to not feeling overwhelmed: support from family and friends and the right problem-solving tools.

GETTING SUPPORT FROM FAMILY
AND FRIENDS

Since other people are not dealing with the person daily, it is normal for them to misunderstand what is going on. Alzheimer's disease is frightening. When people are afraid, they shy away from confronting the truth; they tend to criticize. You may be told the problem is too little mental stimulation; Dad should be stuffed with vitamin B. You may be pressured to choose a nursing home when you do not want to, or relatives and friends may berate you for choosing this option, not understanding that it may be the best choice.

Another natural reaction to fear is to beat a hasty retreat. Relatives no longer call; friends don't come around. Understand that anxiety—not lack of interest—is probably driving them away. If you want their support and involvement, enlighten them. Send articles that explain the disease (see the end of the chapter for some excellent ones); more important, consider inviting family and friends to visit and see what is going on. While you may want to shield other people from "the bitter truth," a dose of reality is unlikely to be much worse than what they are already imagining.

Visits may perk up the person you are caring for, too. Even if you think your husband is too confused to know or get any pleasure from the grandchildren, you might be surprised. We all can guess, but we never know exactly what glimmers of understanding remain in anyone's mind.

Or if visiting is genuinely too threatening, educate loved ones and help them rally around via a more formal route. If your doctor is involved and knowledgeable, ask him to set up a family meeting to explain the illness. Coming from a neutral third party, your need for support and understanding will penetrate loud and clear. You may be surprised how even alienated family members may reach out in sympathy once they understand what you are coping with.

PROBLEM-SOLVING STRATEGIES

Because the behavior this disease produces can be so difficult, every person caring for a dementia victim sometimes feels at loose ends. But people who actively work at solving problems are better off than those who just throw up their hands. While handling alarming symptoms is hard, it is a skill that can be learned.

Psychologist Steve Zarit and his colleagues[29] devised these steps to help caregivers find workable solutions to problems that might otherwise leave them gnashing their teeth. Though it is much better to have a trained counselor help you, you might try this approach on your own.

Identify the reasons for the behavior. The best way to do this is to keep a log recording the upsetting behavior, when it happens, your reaction, and anything else relevant to understanding its cause. For instance, your log might read: (1) "Those same questions a million times an hour"—"Happens after I have left her; worst nights when I leave for the day—Attention-getting mechanism? Way of keeping me in the room? Attempt to entertain me?" (2) "Night wandering"—"Worst when she has not gone out during the day. Sure to happen if she takes a nap."

List several possible solutions. Brainstorm, coming up with several ways of stopping the behavior. Some solutions should flow logically from what you have noted in the log. For instance, if you are grappling with problem 1, you might write: "(1) When I go out for the day, I'll ask Mary to come over. (2) Would it be so bad to take her on some of those trips? (3) Look into a day hospital so she won't be so lonely on the days I do go out." If you are struggling with problem 2, this might be your strategy: "(1) Never let her nap during the day! (2) Ask the doctor about changing that sleep-inducing medicine from after lunch to before bed. (3) Take an evening walk with her."

Arrive at a best plan. Evaluate how feasible each solution is, weeding out alternatives that are less likely to work: "It would be hard to keep her with me or always invite people in; the day hospital seems the best choice." "I cannot hover around to prevent her dozing off, but we might both enjoy a brisk evening walk."

Carry out the plan in fantasy. Mentally walk through the

plan to anticipate and get around possible roadblocks: "This is the way I will go about finding a day hospital and getting her in. I will sell her on the idea by methods X, Y, and Z so she doesn't reject it out of hand."

Carry out the plan in reality. Then act. If your plan doesn't work, try another. Do not conclude that what is happening is uncontrollable—that you cannot change things.

Zarit emphasizes that sometimes modifying your feelings may be the answer, even if the person's actions do not change. Behavior tends to be hardest to tolerate when it appears premeditated—when someone seems to be annoying or difficult on purpose.

The thing that drives me up the wall about caring for Mom is that her mind could be better if she tried more. Some days she seems almost herself; the next day she can't remember the simplest thing. On her bad days I sometimes feel like shaking her. I know her mind is better than that! She just seems to be giving up.

When abilities fluctuate, the natural interpretation is that the person could do better with some real effort. Not true! For unknown physiological reasons, people with dementia have good and bad days. Another intensely irritating symptom that merely appears premeditated is insulting accusations. If your wife who has Alzheimer's disease accuses you of stealing her money or her keys, remind yourself her real target is not you. Seeing you as the villain protects her from admitting the unthinkable: "I am losing my grip on life."

When you are confronted with upsetting behavior, school yourself in this idea: the *illness* is responsible. People with dementia cannot help how they act.

UTILIZING EVERY POSSIBLE RESOURCE

Take full advantage of any formal service your community offers. You are not shirking your responsibility. You do not love the person less. Research shows outside help enables people to do a more loving, effective job.[30] Ask your local office of the aging or ADRDA chapter for help in finding these services.

Home health care. A trained attendant or housekeeper comes into your home.

Day centers or hospitals. Your relative attends a center that may offer meals, recreation, rehabilitation, medical services, and social activities. Some day programs are specifically for people with dementia; some are mixed, accepting both people with dementing illnesses and those with purely physical disabilities.

Respite care. The person is periodically admitted to a hospital or other residential setting to allow you some time off.

Family support groups. Family members regularly meet to share information, offer one another support, and solve problems.

Individual counseling. A person trained in dealing with dementia offers guidance in dealing with your loved one.

Because home care, day care, and respite care are for people with any disabling illness, I will discuss these services more fully in the next chapter. Read the information there with this caution in mind: because of the special management problems they present, these options may be less widely available to people with dementia. Increasingly, however, the services are there. Do not be put off if your relative is rejected by one program. Keep looking for another source of help.

Search out these possibilities even if you are handling everything beautifully now. There may come a time when outside help can mean the difference between having to put your loved one in a nursing home and being able to manage at home. This also applies to the last two choices—help for you. Joining an Alzheimer's family support group or seeing a counselor does not mean you are having mental problems. Researchers find that people who avail themselves of these services are less depressed and have a more positive relationship with the person they are caring for.[31]

EXPLORING INSTITUTIONAL CARE

Finding out your options sooner rather than later also includes looking into nursing homes. Know the best nursing homes in your area and perhaps get your relative on some waiting lists even if you vow this is a choice you will never exercise. You may discover that far from being a hated last resort, eventually a nursing home may be absolutely the best choice.

Turn to chapter 10 for guidance on selecting a nursing home. In addition to the considerations I spell out there, evaluate how well any prospective home serves residents with dementia (estimated to be a good 50 percent of the nursing-home population anyway). Nursing homes generally have "orientation" boards with the date, weather, season, and institution's name to help confused residents. Look beyond this minimum. Ask whether there are special activities and services for confused residents. Is there a dementia unit? Are the staff members trained to understand and work with patients who have Alzheimer's disease? Does the home employ mental health professionals? How does the staff handle common problems the disease causes—wandering, agitation, incontinence? Though these services tend to be more expensive, the ideal is to find an institution with a showplace dementia unit, one offering special services and programs for Alzheimer's victims and caring, trained personnel.

If someone you are close to has this devastating illness, use this chapter as a starting point. Thoroughly educate yourself by joining the ADRDA and reading the books suggested on the next pages. It is far from certain that your loved one will have every distressing symptom I have discussed. Some people deteriorate to a point and then stabilize mentally. Others never need nursing-home care. But as Barry Reisberg, a psychiatrist authority, advises, at least until we find a cure for this dreadful illness, you should "hope for the best and plan for the worst." The cliché "knowledge is power" also applies. The more you know, the easier it will be to bear even the worst.

For More Information

ORGANIZATIONS

Alzheimer's Disease and Related Disorders Association, National Headquarters, 70 East Lake Street, Chicago, Illinois 60601 (800) 621–0379; Illinois: (800) 572–6037.
Joining this organization is a must for anyone dealing with a loved one who has a dementing illness. Begun by concerned family

members and with an advisory board of the top researchers in the field, the ADRDA has chapters across the country that offer families information and help. It supports research into the causes, treatment, and cure of Alzheimer's disease and related disorders, provides help to families, sponsors workshops, and lobbies for better legislation affecting victims and their relatives.

The National Institute on Aging, Bethesda, Maryland 20892 (301) 496–1752.

Sponsors research and training on all aspects of aging including dementia. Call for information about the qualifications of researchers, for the activities of the specially designated Alzheimer's disease centers, and for informational brochures about the illness.

(Your local office of the aging will also either have a formal referral and counseling service or offer more information.)

BOOKLETS, PAMPHLETS, AND ARTICLES

Alzheimer's Disease: A Description of the Illness for the Family and Friends of Patients with this Disorder. Chicago: Alzheimer's Disease and Related Disorders Association, 1985.

This short free pamphlet is good for educating people, since it offers basic facts about the illness. Write or call the ADRDA (see above) for copies.

Bylinsky, G. "Medicine's Next Marvel: The Memory Pill," *Fortune,* January 20, 1986.

Excellent article on the latest biochemical research on stimulating memory and treating dementia chemically.

Health Advancement Services. *Family Handbook on Alzheimer's Disease.* New York: Health Advancement Services, 1982.

Though some of this material is somewhat dated, this is an excellent short guide for families of dementia victims. It describes symptoms, course of the illness, and research into causes and focuses heavily on caregiving—how to take care of the person at home, community and institutional alternatives, legal issues, and so on.

Mace, N. L., and P. V. Rabins. *The Thirty-Six Hour Day.* Baltimore: Johns Hopkins University Press, 1985.

The classic guide for caregivers of Alzheimer's disease patients, offering hundreds of practical tips about handling behavior, community alternatives, and other relevant issues.

National Institute on Aging. *Progress Report on Alzheimer's Disease.* Vol. 2; idem, *Alzheimer's Disease: A Scientific Guide for Health Practitioners.* Rockville, Md.: NIA, 1984.

The first booklet describes research on dementia, and the second is a guide for doctors, social workers, and other health-care professionals whose specialty is not dementia. Both are free and are good for a more technical description of new research (and diagnostic approaches). Write or call the National Institute on Aging Public Affairs Office, Room 6C10, Federal Building, 7550 Wisconsin Avenue, Bethesda, Maryland 20892 for copies.

Roach, M. *Another Name for Madness.* Boston: Houghton-Mifflin, 1985.

Beautifully written firsthand account of the author's experiences in dealing with her mother, who had Alzheimer's disease. To get a true flavor of what this illness is really like, this is essential reading.

Zarit, S., N. Orr, and J. Zarit. *The Hidden Victims of Alzheimer's Disease: Families under Stress.* New York: New York University Press, 1985.

This book is for health-care professionals but is also of interest to caregivers. Describes family emotions, individual counseling for caregivers, and family support groups. Read for a professional's view of the issues involved in helping families cope.

10

DISABILITY
AND
HEALTH CARE

My mother had arthritis and pains in her chest when she exerted herself. She also had diabetes. She sometimes got dizzy and had to lie down. The doctor said these were typical problems of old age and she should take it easy. Nothing could be done medically.

In the past few years things have rapidly gone downhill. First she walked with trouble, then some days she couldn't walk at all. She began taking to her bed, often for days at a time. She could no longer cook. She sometimes had accidents because she couldn't get to the toilet in time.

It was clear she needed help. We had the money, so we got a companion from ten to five. Then she fell getting out of bed one night, and we realized someone was needed around the clock. But we never felt secure. She accused the night nurse of mistreating her. We didn't know whether to believe her or not. We wondered and worried. Are the chest pains she says she has today real? Should we call the doctor this time? Is the homemaker stealing her money? Is she pushing her to get dressed or letting her lie in bed all day?

A month ago we moved her to a nursing home. At prices more expensive than a four-star hotel, the round-the-clock companions were eating up all the money. We put her on the waiting list for a home that had been highly recommended, and a bed came through. We agonized. Either act now or put it off. If we passed up this chance we might not have another for months. But the idea of Mom's being in a home was unbearable too.

At ninety-three she is striking—tall, elegant. She looks beautiful even in her nightgown with her hair unbrushed and no makeup on. We were frightened of her being there with the others—the ones who scream all day. Would she be neglected or abused? Would she be able to come to terms with where she was?

We are surprised at how well things have turned out. At Sterling Heights there is a reason to get out of bed. There are things to do during the day. She has taken over helping some of the residents who are worse off than she is. With the hospital steps away, she is not so worried about her chest pains. I'm not saying her life is wonderful (How can it be for someone who can barely get around?) but she is better off now than before. Have nursing homes been given an unfair press?

The road that can have a nursing home as its final stop begins with chronic disease, those illnesses of aging that begin insidiously, get progressively worse, and strike more and more of us as the years advance.

Most older people have at least one chronic illness. However, the medical diagnosis is not the only thing that counts. What is especially important is whether a person's illness causes disability. Chronic diseases set us on the path to a nursing home only when they become severe enough to limit how we function—when they make it difficult to live independently. Although four out of every five people over sixty-five have at least one chronic condition, only about one in five is disabled by illness in even a minor way—an estimated 5.2 million people as of 1985.[1] A much smaller number, 4 percent of women and 3 percent of men, are severely impaired—housebound or confined to bed by chronic disease.

As figure 6 shows, decade by decade an increasing proportion of people fall prey to severe disabilities. However, it is only by our mid-eighties that we run a real risk of being extremely incapacitated by chronic disease. And there is an interesting sex difference: older women are more at risk than older men. The reason is that men are more likely to suffer from chronic diseases that end in death (such as coronary

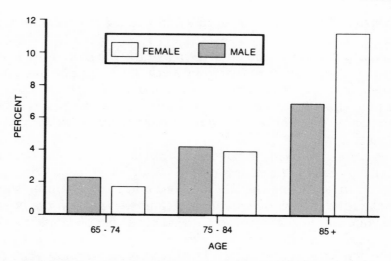

Figure 6   Percentage of people with severe activity limitation, 1982

heart disease), while women are more prone to develop conditions that do not kill but can limit independent living for years (such as osteoporosis).

How important is the distinction between disease and disability to health in the elderly? According to a 1984 report, very important.[2] Among a group of frail older people, researchers found that their subjects' ability to function—manual dexterity, grip strength, walking skill—predicted the chance of imminent nursing-home placement more accurately than traditional medical tests such as assessments of illness based on a physical examination.[3] This study underlines the need to go beyond the standard illness-oriented approach in measuring health in older people. In addition to diagnosing "arthritis" or "heart disease" in an eighty-year-old, another important question should be, How does that diagnosis affect the person's ability to negotiate life?

And understanding health in older people requires another mental shift—from worrying only about life-threatening chronic illnesses (cancer, heart disease, stroke), to viewing diseases that people do not die from as very important too. Though they lack the drama of being potentially fatal, osteoporosis, hearing and vision problems, and arthritis markedly affect the quality of life in our later years. For instance, of the top four disabling chronic diseases in the elderly—heart disease, hypertensive disease, hearing deficits, and arthritis—only the first two pose any threat to life.

So disability is the real old-age enemy, a foe that, while inextricably tied to chronic disease, is not the same thing as "illness" itself. Fighting disability requires a new approach. Doctors have to diagnose and treat "infirmity" as well as the underlying illness; they must widen their focus from life-threatening illnesses to diseases that do not kill but may be just as likely to take us down the path to a nursing home. How well is the medical profession doing at adopting this new approach?

The Doctor's Contribution to Poor Care

According to T. Franklin Williams, director of the National Institute on Aging, it is only recently that doctors have begun to make this shift, tailoring geriatric research and practice to keeping disability at bay.[4] The reorientation has been emotionally difficult because it flies in the face of traditional medicine, which has always been based on a different approach: physicians diagnose an underlying illness, make a brief medical intervention, and hope to effect a dramatic cure.

This single-shot cure-oriented treatment sometimes works with chronic disease, as when a doctor operates to remove cancer or clean out clogged coronary arteries. But in many cases a curative approach is not effective, because most chronic illnesses by definition cannot be cured. Rehabilitation is needed to deal with these illnesses of aging, increasing the patient's ability to function given an unchangeable diagnosis, an illness that will never totally go away. Unfortunately, attacking disability involves using techniques that doctors have been trained to see as less important—exercise, improved nutrition, physical therapy, psychological help, and changing the person's environment to make getting around easier. In addition, these treatments must be chronic too, undertaken for life. And because they cannot make an older body new but can only halt the downward march to a nursing home, they are less exciting than producing a magical, lifesaving cure.

According to Williams, adopting this new approach has also been difficult for many doctors because it means sharing their authority. Social workers, nurses, physical therapists, and dietitians all have vital roles in rehabilitative care.

How important is it for doctors to genuinely collaborate with these lower-status health-care workers in treating older people? According to the findings of this study Williams describes, extremely important. Several teams made up of a physician, a nurse, and dietitian were formed to treat the large group of diabetic residents in a nursing home. Each group met regularly to review its cases and make treatment decisions. Videotapes of the sessions showed that the doctors on the various teams differed markedly in their ability to share decision making with the other group members. In some groups the doctor always had to have the final say. Others were run much more democratically; the doctor was able to see the other group members as true colleagues.

The quality of the care patients received turned out to be directly related to a doctor's leadership style. Doctors who were able to really collaborate with their fellow team members had patients who were healthier and less incapacitated by their disease.

Williams also cautions against another blind spot that doctors tend to have: giving up on older patients.

My doctor wants to get rid of me. Last time I made an appointment because my leg hurt when I walk down steps, and he gave my complaint one minute at the most. He wrote a prescription and rushed me out. I wanted a more thorough examination. Maybe he could have done something for what is wrong. Would there have been a way to deal with the problem without doping myself up? Is there anything I could do on my own that would help? I think it's because I'm eighty and he feels what I have is not worth his time.

People frequently complain that because they are older, their doctors give them short shrift. Unfortunately, scientific evidence supports their claim. About a decade ago researchers at the Rand Corporation clocked the average amount of time physicians in seven specialties spent in visits with patients of various ages.[5] They found that people over sixty-five were seen for the least amount of time. Whether the doctor was an internist or a cardiologist and whether the visit took place in a private office, hospital, or nursing home, the upsetting result was the same—time spent examining and talking to elderly patients averaged significantly less than for other groups. Considering that after age sixty-five we tend to be in worse health and so should need more time and attention, this is unfair indeed.

Luckily, things are changing. Doctors are becoming aware of their attitudes. They are now being trained that we are not powerless in dealing with disabling chronic disease. Within the past fifteen years the number of medical schools offering courses in geriatrics has grown from a handful to a majority. By 1995 experts estimate that every medical school will offer at least some training in this exciting new field.[6] Here is some of the information that geriatrics courses provide.

Diseases can produce different symptoms in older people than they do in the young. An interesting example is a heart attack. In younger people its wrenching pain is impossible to miss. But by our seventies the only sign of a heart attack may be mental confusion or indigestion.[7] Earlier, doctors might often have sent an elderly heart attack victim home with antacids. Today's more geriatrically aware physicians are less likely to make this fatal mistake.

Age does not equal illness. In geriatrics courses doctors learn that not all older people are sick. In fact, as we grow older we differ more and more from one another physically (see chap. 1). Students are taught to view their older patients as individuals, not as bodies aged eighty or ninety-five.

What physical changes are normal and what are pathological. Geriatric training makes doctors sensitive about labeling the many things that can be helped as just "old age." They are less likely to overtreat too, reading illness into normal changes or pushing drugs excessively. By learning about studies such as the Baltimore study sponsored by the National Institute on Aging, they get a better sense of when to treat their patients and when not to intervene.

To restore function. They are also trained in the orientation toward disability I just described: improving eighty-year-old

Mrs. Jones's ability to get around can be as worthwhile a goal as curing her disease. If she can get to the store, she may not have to move. She can continue to live with her husband and will not have the heartbreak of going to a nursing home. Reaching these goals may mean arranging for a physical therapist to come to her home to increase her mobility and strength; knowing about the many gadgets that can make life easier for the disabled; treating the depression that is compounding her physical problems; working with her family; knowing what community services are available to keep people out of nursing homes.

The Patient's Contribution to Poor Care

Unfortunately, in spite of this new focus on geriatrics, there is unhappy evidence that many doctors today still may be giving their older patients less attention.[8] In a 1987 study, when researchers videotaped the doctor/patient interviews of five typical private-practice physicians, they discovered that with older people doctors tended to focus on physical symptoms alone. Conversations about the effects of the illness—whether the patient was having trouble getting around and was worried or depressed—were much more likely to take place with younger adults.

However, the patients seemed as much at fault as the doctors. During their visits, elderly people brought up only their dizziness, or pain, or blood pressure. Younger patients tended to raise a broader set of questions, focusing both on their symptoms and on how their illness was affecting their lives.

So when older people are given less attention, they themselves may be partly to blame. Being trained in the idea that the doctor is an authority figure, they may be less aggressive in bringing up their concerns. Because they demand less from their doctors, they get less.

Sociologist Marie Haug of Case Western Reserve University, who has done extensive research on elderly patient/physician relationships, finds older people are also guilty of therapeutic pessimism and are just as prone to self-diagnose treatable conditions as old age.[9] Because not feeling well is supposed to be "normal" at age seventy or eighty, many people are reluctant to call their doctors when a symptom appears. Their attitude is, "At my age what can any doctor do?"

My hand has begun shaking uncontrollably, and my wife tells me I should give the doctor a call. I'm reluctant. After all, I'm seventy-eight. It's not like the shaking is so bad. I can walk. I can play golf. My life is not in danger. When I look around, I see how bad things could be. I don't need to be in a nursing home. I don't have heart trouble. I'm better off than most men my age. Why should a person in the pink of health waste the doctor's time?

This reasoning condemns people to live with what they have; they lose the race by default, neglecting to put in a bet. When this man was badgered into making an appointment, his doctor prescribed a far from painful remedy—a drink of Scotch a day. He now takes his "medicine" each evening, and his shaking is gone.

Many symptoms that seem to be old age are treatable. Even real age-related disabilities—such as problems in walking or dressing—often can improve. When gerontologists at Ohio State University traced the course of disabilities like these in several thousand older men over a fifteen-year period from 1966 to 1981, they found that more of us do develop infirmities as the years advance, but disabilities also go away. Many men who had trouble reaching, lifting, or walking in 1976 did not have the same problems five years later in 1981.[10] What looks like the permanent physical ravages of aging can be surprisingly temporary.

Furthermore, a 1986 report shows that rehabilitation can work wonders. When 190 severely disabled older people were treated at a special geriatric rehabilitation center, the changes were dramatic. The number who could function on their own (at least partially) increased from 87 to 173. Those able to walk independently rose from 42 to 127.[11]

Getting High-Quality Medical Care

The success rate of this program shows that to wage war against disabilities it is important to have high-quality medical care. Here are some ways to help ensure you get that care.

HANDLING THE PHYSICIAN/PATIENT
RELATIONSHIP

School yourself in the modern point of view. You and your physician are collaborators. The doctor is obliged to treat you as an intelligent person, to explain things to you carefully in understandable terms. You have the obligation to want to know and should take the following steps to be a responsive partner in your care.

Call your doctor when you experience any unusual new symptom or physical change. It is not necessary to pick up the phone at every headache or cold, but when anything *unusual* happens physically, give your doctor a call. If thoughts like these give you pause—"It's old age"; "I don't want to bother the doctor"; "He can't do anything for me"—tell yourself, "Until I get my medical degree, I'll let Dr. Jones be the judge."

Visit or call armed with a written list of questions. Many people get flustered when they talk to a doctor and forget half of what they wanted to say. So be organized. Write down every question before you see your physician. Make your list as comprehensive as possible. Understand that difficulties such as getting to the store are also legitimate problems for the doctor to help you with.

Ask for exact information about what tests, treatments, and diagnoses mean. Do not accept "doctorese." Insist on explanations you can understand. When the doctor prescribes drugs, know what to expect and what the possible side effects are (see chap. 1). When your physician suggests surgery, know the risks and the nonsurgical alternatives.

Question your doctor thoroughly if anything is unclear. Squelch the thought, "She's too busy" or "I'm being difficult." Take all the time you need. If you still have doubts or questions after you leave the office, get more information. Don't hesitate to call back armed with a new list.

If necessary, read about your problem on your own. Go to a library and check out some medical books. You may not have gone to medical school, but any intelligent person can become a lay expert in an area of special concern.

Report side effects of medications or treatments promptly. If a prescribed drug makes you feel bad, rather than suffering in silence or not following through, call back. Your doctor may be able to suggest an alternative treatment that works without having the side effect.

When surgery is recommended, get other opinions. Medicare will pay for any surgical second opinion and also pays the full cost of a third if the first two doctors disagree. To get a second opinion, rather than asking for a name from the specialist who recommended the operation, call your family doctor for a referral. Or call the national toll-free Second Opinion Hotline: (800) 638–6833. This Medicare-operated service gives anyone who calls the name of a local agency that maintains a list of doctors in the area who have agreed to give second opinions. Then call your county medical society to learn the qualifications of the physician suggested. They will have information about the credentials and affiliations of every licensed doctor in your area.

Or try this approach: call a top-rated teaching hospital and ask for an appointment with the chairman of the department that handles your disease (the chief of cardiology, oncology, etc.). If you cannot see that person, ask for a referral to another senior faculty member. For your own peace of mind, try to get any second opinion about surgery from the very best source.

Since some of these suggestions may be difficult to implement on your own, consider asking a relative or close friend to help. Could your brash son-in-law be prevailed on to set up an appointment with that ultracompetent, hard-to-reach specialist? On your monthly visits to the doctor, could your daughter or Mrs. Smith from around the corner accompany you? Because things move so quickly during those often-rushed office visits, having a companion (that is, an ally) to step in and slow things down may increase the chance that your concerns will be heard. Meet beforehand to formulate your list of concerns and questions. And check with one another before you leave the office: "Was anything Dr. Jones said unclear?" "Do I have other things to ask?"

EVALUATING YOUR CURRENT PHYSICIAN

Unfortunately, few doctors now practicing have been trained in geriatrics. But good physicians will have intuitively learned to adapt their approach to the special needs of patients who are older or disabled by chronic disease. Before age even enters the equation, your doctor must have the twin essentials for providing good care—technical competence and a good bedside manner.

A good bedside manner is not irrelevant to quality treatment. We are more likely to visit a doctor who is warm and accepting; we are more likely to make an appointment and to follow through on any procedure the doctor suggests. Having a doctor with a congenial personality is even more important as we grow older, because our physicians are almost destined to become much more central in our lives. These 1983 statistics are a grim testament: in that year, Americans aged twenty-five to forty-four saw a doctor an average of 4.8 times; the figure for people over seventy-five was 8.4 times.[12]

Dealing with chronic illnesses involves ongoing collaboration. It behooves you to have a collaborator who seems caring, whom you can talk to honestly, who values what you say, who believes that something can be done for you, whom you can feel free to "bother" with any reasonable question or concern.

On the other hand, a pleasing personality can be seductive. We tend to develop an intense attachment to our doctors, a combination of respect and adoration very like the bond young children develop with their parents. We are especially likely to develop these "transference" feelings if we have a long-standing relationship with our doctors, are seeing them regularly, and have a potentially fatal disease. But love can blind, and blind loyalty can be dangerous. It can cause us to put up with poor care beyond the time we should. We don't get a second opinion because we are afraid it will hurt the doctor. We have been with him for thirty years, and he has always treated us so well. We may be afraid if we change doctors we will not get the same attention. "Won't I lose my special relationship with Dr. Smith if he learns I consulted someone else?"

My husband is assertive in his business, but he is jelly when it comes to saving his own life. He has cancer of the throat. The prognosis is not good. I know oncologists differ in their skill and their ability to cure. He insists on staying with the first

*doctor we consulted, a man I know is second-rate. I think an-
other doctor might be his life raft, or at least buy him more
time. He is clinging like a baby to this sinking ship.*

If you suspect you are getting inadequate care, harden your
heart. Put aside loyalty, love, and inertia and get a consultation. What you learn may make you more secure, or you may
discover your suspicions are right—that you must steel yourself and find a new doctor.

SELECTING A NEW DOCTOR

Changing doctors is an unpleasant task that many older people face, not just the few who awaken to the fact that their
trusted family physicians are less than competent. You may
have moved after retirement. Or you and your doctor may
have grown old together. One year he decides to retire. It is
hard to start again from scratch after losing a relationship that
may have spanned much of your adult life. You may feel no
one will know your body in the same way. Never again will
you get the same special attention or care.

These fears are natural. Anyone we have such an intimate
relationship with for so long is bound to seem irreplaceable.
The truth is that transference is transferable. Provided you
make a determined search, you can find a doctor you will
eventually feel just as enthusiastic about. But you must
choose wisely. Make selecting a replacement a special project.
What other investment of time is more important?[13] (Once
again, it may be helpful to enlist another person in following
the next suggestions, a competent "buddy" who can work
with you—or even take over the job—in making this project
succeed.)

Develop a list of names. Question friends and relatives, but
give most weight to recommendations by doctors or other
health-care professionals. They will be better able to evaluate
candidates' skills. You can feel more confident that someone
they suggest is competent, not just affable.

Check the credentials of each person on your list. What
training and education does the doctor have? Does he or she
have an academic appointment at a medical school? What hos-

pital is the physician affiliated with, and what is its reputation? To get these facts, either call the doctor's office directly or ask your county medical society.

Expense. Find out the doctor's fees and when payments are due. If your financial situation is tight, would it be possible to arrange a special payment schedule to fit your budget? Find out if the doctor accepts Medicare (or if you are eligible, Medicaid), and if so, for what services. Will the office bill Medicare and your insurance carrier directly?

Medicare will pay only for the services of licensed physicians. Your doctor may bill Medicare directly, or you may pay and then be reimbursed by Medicare. Whatever arrangement you have with your doctor, after you pay the yearly deductible, Medicare pays 80 percent of what it deems the "reasonable charge," and you pay the other 20 percent. *If your doctor charges more than the "reasonable charge," you are responsible for the additional amount.*

If feasible, choose a doctor who takes what is called "Medicare assignment." This means that even if his normal fee is higher, he agrees not to charge you more than Medicare will cover. Those who accept Medicare assignment also submit claim forms directly to Medicare, which will save you time. Unfortunately, however, it is increasingly hard to find a doctor who does accept assignment. Because of Medicare's stingy reimbursement rates, nationwide 72 percent do not.

Accessibility. Find out if the office is close by or near public transportation. Will it be easy to get there if your health changes for the worse? Assess how easy it will be to reach the doctor. What are the office hours, and what is the policy if an emergency occurs after hours? Is another doctor on call when yours is unavailable?

If the doctor is part of a group practice, the associates will cover. Doctors in solo practice generally make arrangements with another practitioner to take their calls when they are away. Be as sure as possible that you will be able to get immediate attention when you need it.

Answers to these questions will help narrow your choices. When you visit, look for the following signs.

Quality of the services. Is the doctor prompt, or are you kept waiting for hours? Is the office clean and well equipped? Are you given a thorough examination?

On this first visit, expect the doctor to spend a good deal of time reviewing your medical history. Be prepared to discuss everything important—your major illnesses and operations, the drugs you regularly take, bad reactions to past treatments, any allergies or sensitivities. Get a sense of whether the doctor is questioning you fully and giving you ample time to talk. In the physical examination, the same considerations apply. Is this someone who seems careful and competent? Is this a person you feel comfortable with and can trust?

Look for signs of geriatric sensitivity. Does the doctor dismiss symptoms that bother you as "old age"? Do you get the feeling that what you say is being discounted because you are over seventy-five? Does this person seem to prescribe drugs precipitously? Are you carefully questioned about the medications you are taking now?

If you have a chronic disease, the doctor should be concerned about how your condition is affecting your ability to function and knowledgeable about the total approach to care discussed earlier—rehabilitation, supportive aids, community services. Choose someone who seems interested in more than the strictly physical side of your disease.

THE HMO ALTERNATIVE

Increasingly, rather than selecting a private doctor, you may have another choice—joining a health maintenance organization or HMO. Rather than paying a physician for each appointment, if you join an HMO you pay a fixed sum in advance that entitles you to almost all (or all) of your medical care: checkups and routine care, laboratory tests, the services of specialists, hospitalization costs. There are two major types of HMOs—group practice and individual practice.[14]

Group-practice HMOs provide all their outpatient services at a centrally located health facility, usually staffed by primary-care doctors, specialists (e.g., in eye care, hearing, surgery, gynecology), and additional personnel such as technicians and nurses. The clinic offers laboratories, X-ray services, a pharmacy, and perhaps ambulatory surgical care. On enrolling, a subscriber selects one of the primary-care doctors as a personal physician who is responsible for coordinating care. On routine visits patients may see a specially trained nurse practitioner.

Individual-practice HMOs provide primary care in the private offices of doctors under contract to the HMO. Joining this type of HMO may make getting to the doctor easier if you choose someone with an office near your home, but you may not receive the wide range of services you would get by joining a group-practice HMO.

A major advantage of joining an HMO is more financial peace of mind. Your medical bill is already paid. There are no large out-of-pocket expenses you might abruptly incur. There also is no economic deterrent to calling the doctor if you are ill, since visiting four times a month costs no more than once a month. And because HMOs have to operate within a fixed budget, they have an incentive to deliver services in an economical fashion. Studies show that, on average, people who use HMOs spend less for health care.

Does this emphasis on efficiency lead to poorer service? Although doctors opposed to HMOs reason that a system where people are paid beforehand no matter what they do offers a built-in incentive to provide minimal, cursory care, the reverse seems to be true. When researchers at Johns Hopkins Medical School reviewed the literature comparing HMO care with traditional fee-for-service care, nineteen studies showed that HMOs provided better care, a handful found the two types of care comparable, and only one or two found HMO care inferior.[15]

On the other hand, the serious drawback to joining an HMO is the lack of freedom. HMO subscribers must use a certain hospital; when they need a specialist, they must visit someone under contract to the HMO. Many people decide against joining because they are not prepared to give up the right to go to the doctor or hospital of their choice.

Furthermore, only a fraction of HMOs accept Medicare. (Some HMOs not under contract to Medicare provide what is called Medicare "wraparound," offering coverage for current subscribers, who then become eligible for Medicare.) Probably in part because of this, only a small minority of the elderly are enrolled in HMOs.

If you are interested in an HMO and able to enroll, use the same considerations in evaluating it as you would in selecting a private physician: cost (Does the HMO accept Medicare? How expensive is joining? What services are covered?); accessibility (How easy is it to get there? Will a doctor see you promptly if you are ill?); quality (Is the clinic overcrowded and unattractive? Are the doctors on the staff well qualified? What is the affiliated hospital like?).

James Doherty of the Group Health Association of America, a national organization of HMOs, also suggests finding out if the HMO is "federally qualified." Federally qualified HMOs are approved by the Health Care Financing Administration. Your state insurance department will also have information about the quality of a prospective HMO.[16]

WHEN TO CHOOSE A GERIATRIC SPECIALIST

As long as you select someone who seems aware of your needs, your physician need not have formal training in geriatrics. If you have several disabling conditions or are in your eighties or beyond and need to change doctors, however, it makes sense to search out a geriatric specialist. If a doctor has been recommended as specializing in geriatrics, find out exactly what training he or she has had. Ask about plans to take the newly developed licensing examination in the field.

If you live in an urban area, explore the possibility of getting care from a hospital-based geriatric service. Geriatric services offer state-of-the-art team care for disabled older people—workers from a variety of disciplines collaborate to keep people functioning independently. If this type of service is available, the care is likely to be excellent. You will be surprised at the attention and the sensitivity to your needs. People committed to geriatrics are a special breed; they combine technical skill with heart. When necessary, they are even happy to make house calls.

Another alternative you may have is a freestanding geriatric center. To understand what services this type of institution can provide, let's examine the offerings of one—the Metropolitan Jewish Geriatric Center in Brooklyn, New York.

The Metropolitan Jewish Geriatric Center provides what it calls an "umbrella approach" to geriatric care, addressing the full spectrum of needs of older people who are having some trouble functioning independently. It offers inpatient services and a variety of outpatient programs. There is long-term home health care for people who are housebound: all the nursing, rehabilitation, and medical services of a nursing home are offered in a patient's own home. There is the day hospital, a center open from nine to five offering activities, meals, nursing, and rehabilitation. There is the hospice program for people who are terminally ill. (Hospices minister to dying patients and their families, offering counseling and treatment directed toward pain control and comfort rather than cure. To enter this program, now covered by Medicare, a person must be judged as having no more than six months to live and must be willing to abandon curative treatments.) There also is an Emergency Alarm Response System (EARS). For a small monthly charge a subscriber's telephone is hooked up to a central switchboard. Someone calls daily to check in. If there is no answer, a neighbor comes by to check. The older person living alone has the comfort of knowing help will arrive in a medical emergency.[17]

There also is Elderplan, an HMO specifically for people over sixty-five. By paying a fixed sum, enrollees are entitled to all the outpatient services the center offers plus traditional medical and hospital care and care in a nursing home.

Except for Elderplan, all the programs offered at this geriatric center are now available in many communities. They are components of what is called a continuum of care. They exist to prevent nursing-home placement, to keep people with disabilities functioning in the community.

The rest of this chapter is intended for family members dealing with a disabled older relative. What community services should you be considering? What if the answer must be a nursing home?

Community Alternatives to Nursing Homes

When people begin to have trouble with cooking or getting around and their families cannot care for them, the knee-jerk reaction is to consider *just* a nursing home. But a nursing home may not be needed. Surveys show that some nursing-home residents do not need to be institutionalized; they could live in the community if they took advantage of the outpatient alternatives that exist. For instance, in one demonstration project, people otherwise bound for nursing homes called a special triage number. Through the use of community resources, the health-care team operating the project was able to keep 25 to 30 percent of these callers at home.[18]

The decision to put a loved one in a nursing home frequently is made after a medical crisis. The patient is in a hospital and must be discharged soon. Handling life at home right now is impossible. There is a mad scramble to find a nursing-home bed. There is no time to explore other possibilities or even to select the best nursing home.

But in a hospital people are at their physical worst. After they recuperate they may not need institutional care. They may require only minor help with shopping or cooking or getting around. Placing this type of person in a nursing home is like using a sledgehammer to treat a problem that could be cured by a tap. And it is physically wasteful. Offering too much care produces excess disabilities, further eroding the quality of life.

A comparison of patients who entered nursing homes and two other groups with similar disabilities receiving different types of home care underlines this point. After three months the patients getting care in the community made greater improvements in their ability to care for themselves and get around, and they were happier than the group in the nursing homes.[19]

Nursing-home care can also be financially wasteful. It is very expensive, costing on the average $20,000 to $25,000 a year. Medicare covers *1 percent* of the cost.[20] The Medicare system covers only acute or curative care. Once care is labeled as custodial, chronic, or forever, Medicare will not pay.

Although nursing-home insurance has recently become

available, it too is expensive—about $1,500 a year for subscribers in their seventies, more costly beyond that age.[21] A 1987 review of thirty-one policies showed that qualifying for this type of insurance can also be hard. Companies often impose numerous eligibility restrictions—for instance, weeding out anyone with obvious disabilities or even denying coverage if a person answers yes to *any* health-related question on the application. Policies can have numerous "exceptions" or provide very limited coverage for certain types of nursing-home care.[22]

Most people begin by paying the astronomical nursing-home fees privately. In fact, while a mere 5 percent of people over sixty-five are residents of nursing homes, the lion's share of the out-of-pocket health-care dollar spent each year by this age group goes not to hospitals or physicians, but to nursing homes (see fig. 7). The steep expense bankrupts all but the wealthiest; resources are soon exhausted, and the nursing-home resident becomes eligible for Medicaid, the health-care insurance system for the poor, which does cover custodial care. This scenario fits an estimated half-million people every year.[23]

If a relative is having problems functioning independently, you should explore every alternative to a nursing home. Visit your local office for the aging for information about what exists in your community. Get a full consultation from a social worker on the staff. Even when the answer must be a nursing home, the judicious use of these services may buy you time— to search out the best nursing home, to allow your relative to share the decision making and absorb the news, to make the transition to institutional living less wrenching.

The community services described below can also be costly. But unless full-time home care is required, they are likely to be much less expensive than paying privately for a nursing home. Just as Medicare covers only services defined as "rehabilitative or curative" in a nursing home, this condition also applies to its paying for noninstitutional care. Unless a service is defined as medical and noncustodial and a doctor certifies that your relative needs it, Medicare is unlikely to pay.

While Medicaid, the health-insurance system for the poor, does cover noninstitutional custodial care, specifically what it

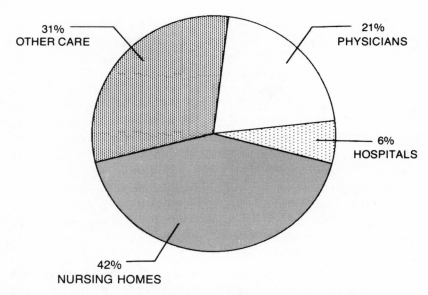

Figure 7   Where the out-of-pocket dollar for the elderly goes, 1984. Notice the exorbitant bill for home care and nursing home care.

will pay for varies from state to state—the reason being that whereas Medicare is federally administered, the Medicaid program is under the jurisdiction of individual states. Here are the services to consider.

HOME CARE

Home care is the most widespread alternative to nursing-home care, a spectrum of services involving everything from round-the-clock skilled nursing to a few hours' help each week with housekeeping, laundry, and meals. Because of advances in technology, today even people who genuinely need twenty-four-hour skilled nursing can get this type of intensive care in their homes, if they are able to participate in one of the few free demonstration projects for Medicaid recipients or are willing to foot the enormous bill privately. Generally speaking, however, home care, like any community service to forestall institutionalization, is most appropriate for people who do not require the intense services of a nursing home but do need minor to moderate help in negotiating life.

If your relative is being discharged from a hospital, the hospital social worker can help you find appropriate home care. Otherwise, either consult your office of the aging or go it on your own. Look in the Yellow Pages under "nursing care" or "home health care" for an agency. Be guided by these clues to quality—the words "certified" and "accredited."[24]

Certified home health-care agencies are government licensed and are the only ones able to accept Medicare or Medicaid. They provide a variety of home-care workers. Getting an employee from a certified agency is preferable because government regulations specify that anyone the agency sends to your home must have a certain number of hours of training.

Accredited agencies have met even more rigorous standards, requirements set up by nonprofit organizations dedicated to promoting high-quality home care. Accreditation is voluntary and takes place only after a careful review. While an agency may be excellent and still not be accredited, choosing this type of service ensures that you are dealing with the best.

The label *licensed* simply signifies that the agency has met basic legal and operating requirements. Services gotten through licensed, noncertified agencies must be paid for privately. If you decide to use this type of agency, find out how extensively it trains its employees.

In addition to independent agencies, hospitals are increasingly likely to offer home-care services. Or home-care programs may be operated by nursing homes and geriatric centers.

Once you call, the agency should offer you guidance in choosing the right type of care—services fitting your relative's financial and physical requirements (see table 8). When it sends you workers, a good agency will also monitor what is happening and resolve any problems. However, you also have to do your share in demanding quality care.

The front-line home-care workers—homemakers, home health attendants—are not highly paid. There is no prospect of advancement. Their job is often mentally and physically taxing. If possible, make sure the person caring for your relative is experienced, trustworthy, and competent and genuinely likes older people. While you are apt to have to make compromises, ideally you should be searching out someone like this:

Table 8   Home-Care Workers: A Partial List

Social workers
Provide counseling and find, coordinate, and supervise home-care services.

Registered dietitians
Plan special diets to speed recovery from illness or to manage conditions such as diabetes.

Physical therapists
Use exercise, heat, light, water, and such to treat problems of movement.

Occupational therapists
Teach people how to function at their best with disabilities—for example, how to do housework from a wheelchair.

Nurses
RNs (registered nurses) provide skilled nursing care; LPNs (licensed practical nurses) offer simpler nursing services. The former are more highly trained and are needed mainly to treat complex medical conditions.

Homemaker/home health aides
Usually the primary caretakers; may do cleaning, housekeeping, bathing, dressing, and other types of personal care. Their job title varies considerably, depending in part on the mix of help provided. For example, "homemaker" or "housekeeper" may be the title when the person mainly does cleaning; "home health aide" or "attendant" may be used when personal care is mainly involved.

Chore workers
Assist with services such as yardwork, home repair, or heavy cleaning.

What a relief it was to find Mary when my mother's physical condition was going downhill! She approached her job with a combination of professionalism and genuine love. I felt confident Mom was being treated kindly. And she gently pushed her to get up and dressed and sit outside. When something was wrong, she knew it and could be trusted to give the doctor a call. He said he was amazed at her ability to understand when Mom was really sick.

DAY HOSPITALS AND PROGRAMS

This service, now widely available, is exclusively for people who are able to leave the house. In a day program, your relative goes out to a center (transportation often is also available) where treatment and social activities are offered during the day. Day centers are usually open from 9:00 to 4:00 five days a week, though registrants may vary in the number of days they attend. There are two types.

Day hospitals offer a variety of medical and social activities—nursing help, physical and occupational therapy, and medical supervision as well as recreation (bingo, etc.) and a noon meal. A *social day care* program is nonmedical in focus, usually providing only a meal, recreation, and limited social services.

The cost varies. Day hospitals—because they offer much more—are more expensive than social day care, but Medicare and private insurance may pay for part (Medicaid is likely to pay for more). Social day care is a nonmedical service, so it is not covered by any medical plan, though some programs may have a sliding scale depending on ability to pay.

DECIDING BETWEEN HOME CARE
AND DAY CARE

A day program may be the right alternative if you are worried about the care someone coming to your home might provide. They can offer more peace of mind because of their visibility. There is less chance of mistreatment when so many people are watching than there might be in the privacy of your relative's home. They also offer a more stimulating environment. They may be less costly than one-to-one care. Also, when you choose a day hospital, medical and nursing services are there, lessening the work of orchestrating these visits on your own.

However, in general day care does *not* offer the flexibility of home care. Centers tend to serve a more limited group, people who qualify for the program. Your relative may be barred from a program if there is a change in medical condition or if behavioral problems develop. The hours are more rigid. Services tend to be available only on weekdays. And because patients cannot attend the program during an acute illness, choosing this alternative means being more vulnerable to the need for other arrangements. Because it is even more difficult to go somewhere strange than to have someone strange come in, it also may be harder to convince your loved one to attend a daycare program. So if convenience is a main consideration, home care is a better choice.

RESPITE CARE

This newest and therefore least widespread program is specifically for caregivers, to give them a break from the burden of ministering fulltime to a disabled family member. The person admitted to respite care periodically enters an inpatient setting—generally a nursing home or geriatric center—for several days or longer so family members can go on vacation or have time off. The major disadvantages of respite care are its limited availability and the fact that no health insurance covers it.

SPECIALIZED SERVICES

A variety of more limited services also helps put off the need for a nursing home: home-delivered meals, transportation, shopping assistance, home repair, and telephone systems like that offered by the geriatric center described above. Some of these services may be available free or almost free. Others are offered on a sliding scale of payment.

While your area office on aging is the best general source for what is available, sectarian organizations are a good second choice—Catholic, Protestant, or Jewish. Groups such as the American Heart Association, the Arthritis Foundation, and the Alzheimer's Disease and Related Disorders Association offer advice on disabilities caused by these specific diseases. Or turn to the social work department or geriatric service of your local hospital for help.

MODIFYING THE ENVIRONMENT
TO ENHANCE INDEPENDENCE

Apart from finding out about community services, changing the environment may help. *Shop for items to make life easier.* Are you afraid your mother may fall in the tub? A set of grab bars may be the answer. Are the controls on her stove or her faucets too hard to turn? There may be a gadget that can help. Does it worry you that your father cannot hear the phone? Look for a device that amplifies the sound of the bell or the caller's voice. Even ordering the large print edition of the newspaper can raise your relative's spirits and so increase the distance from a nursing home.

You can find helpful items by visiting a medical supply store or even a hardware store. Or you can send for products listed in the books and catalogs at the end of this chapter. Another place to call is the occupational therapy department of your local hospital. Occupational therapists specialize in rehabilitation. Their job is to know the range of devices and environmental modifications that make life easier for people with disabilities.

You may want to make a more radical environmental modification—convince your relative to move. Would your mother function better if she lived around the corner from you or moved to a smaller apartment? Perhaps you can get her into one of the growing number of residences that offer meals, maid service, and personal care to older people who are having some trouble handling life on their own. (Once again, your local office for the aging is the place to get information on this type of housing.)

When a Nursing Home Is Needed

Sometimes, in spite of exploring every option, the only solution will be a nursing home, as when someone is severely disabled requiring a level of care beyond what the family can provide, and home care is financially or physically impossible.

If your relative is in this situation, try not to view what is happening as a tragedy. Nursing-home placement is far from being a disaster for everyone. In fact research shows that when people are barely hanging on to coping, going to a nursing home tends to be a welcome relief (see chap. 8). My own experience bears this out. During the year I worked in a nursing home I found a good deal of misery, but I also met many residents who were genuinely happy. Some of the most unlikely people flourished in this protected environment.

My mother spent her adult life being pampered; when we had to send her to Four Acres, we knew it would kill her. We did not think she could survive the comedown and the shame. We lived through the agony of our decision and came to terms with our guilt at putting her away. And then there was the happy shock. She is much better off now that she is here! For the first time in years, she is not isolated. She is kept busy and active. She has a reason to put on makeup, to get her hair done. She has taken up painting; because of the daily physical therapy, she can walk by herself again.

Good nursing homes offer a variety of features that home care cannot provide: activities and stimulation, the equipment and personnel for rehabilitation, immediate attention in a medical emergency. There is even research suggesting that nursing-home placement improves family harmony. In one study family members had a more loving relationship with relatives who had entered a home, because the day-to-day worry was gone.[25]

And nursing homes are not just a final holding pattern before death, as a study done at Brown University showed: the researchers found that 26 percent of the residents of the typical nursing home they studied were discharged to the community—most to live independently in their own homes.[26] The patients' prognosis at entry turned out to be the best predictor of their eventual fate. Most people whom doctors expected should be able to return home did. In other words, the pronouncement "this is temporary" is indeed trustworthy.

This is not to paint a false picture. Nursing homes are not basically desirable places to be. Many people deteriorate rapidly after they enter. Some nursing homes richly deserve the description snake pit. However, taking the following steps can help ensure that placement is not a tragedy.

SELECT KNOWLEDGEABLY

Nursing homes are categorized in two definite ways: by the intensity of services they provide and by their mode of ownership. The first distinction is crucial. Medicaid (or Medicare) will pay for services only in nursing homes classified as offering either skilled or intermediate care.

Skilled nursing facilities provide the most care, including round-the-clock nursing, physical, occupational, and dietary therapy, social services, and recreation. *Health-related facilities* (or *intermediate care facilities*) are for people who do not need skilled care but do need some assistance in functioning. They offer less intensive nursing and medical care. *Multilevel facilities* are most common, providing skilled and intermediate care under one roof. The advantage of choosing a multilevel nursing home is that your relative will receive services in the same place (though probably on a different floor or in another building) if there is a change in condition and a different level of care is required.

You cannot choose the level of nursing care when your relative is admitted. The person is placed at the appropriate level by a doctor or nurse certifying eligibility for that particular type. Although the evaluation process tends to differ from state to state, usually a standard preadmission form is required. The person is examined, and points are assigned for degrees of disability. Depending on this "impairment" score, the applicant may be categorized as not needing institutional care, needing a health-related facility, or needing skilled nursing care.

Medicare will pay only for care in a skilled nursing facility, and then only in limited circumstances. Up to one hundred days may be covered if a doctor certifies that the patient requires ongoing nursing care for a condition that was first treated in the hospital and if the nursing home's utilization review committee does not disapprove the stay. *These rules are rigorously applied.* Depending on the state, Medicaid is likely to pay for all or most skilled or intermediate care.

(Check with your local office of the aging or the admissions department of the home you are interested in for more information.)

The second nursing home difference, mode of ownership, is less relevant. *Proprietary homes* are owned and run for a profit. *Voluntary homes* are owned and run by nonprofit organizations such as church groups. *Public homes* are owned by the city or state. Recently there has been a tremendous increase in the number of proprietary chains. There is some perception that these institutions, because they are in the money-making business, tend to deliver worse care. But research shows there is no way to predict the quality of care a home offers by its mode of ownership.[27]

Apart from these distinctions there is bewildering variety. Nursing homes differ by size, religious and ethnic orientation, and philosophy of care. Choosing a home depends on personal preference, your sense of where your relative would do best. For instance, larger homes tend to offer much more in the way of services and a richer variety of staff. They are less homelike, however, getting lower marks on staff/patient rapport.[28] Your choice will also be dictated by the type of residents the home serves. Although the law prohibits discrimination in admission, many nursing homes cater to the needs and comfort of a particular ethnic or religious group—serving familiar foods, celebrating traditional holidays.

Philosophical differences can be important. Does the home believe in separating residents by degree of disability? This may be good if your father is not very impaired and would be depressed by being in close contact with residents who are physically and mentally worse off. It may be bad if he would benefit from being with residents who are more alert. Does the home have a special unit for residents with Alzheimer's disease? If so, this may be the best place for your mother with dementia.

Consider the location. In general, the closer the better, either to you or to your relative's hometown. If the home is near the patient's town, remaining involved in the life of the community may be possible. Your relative's personal doctor may agree to continue treatment. (Residents always have the right to be treated by a physician of their own choice, though they may have to pay extra for this service.) If the home is close to you, you can visit often. You will be better able to offer your love and attention and also to check up on what is going on.

With these considerations in mind, talk to family and friends who know residents in the homes you are considering. Then visit each place. The first time you go, arrive unannounced. Expect what you see to be disheartening. Only people in the worst physical straits need nursing homes. Your first instinct may even be "God forbid I put Mom here!" Force yourself to look beyond its occupants, to consider the home itself. Would your mother profit from what is offered? Are the services of high quality?

Arrive armed with this excellent checklist adapted from *A Consumer Guide to Nursing Home Care in New York City*, put out by a nursing-home advocacy group, the Friends and Relatives of the Institutionalized Aged.[29]

The physical plant. Is the home clean, well lit, relatively odor-free, laid out with a disabled person's needs in mind? Do residents' rooms contain personal belongings? What is the policy on bringing in such belongings? Is there enough room for privacy and an attractive place to sit outside?

You want a place that looks cheerful and is appropriate for people who have problems in walking or seeing or hearing well, where the environment minimizes excess disabilities. You also want an administration that is sensitive to a crucial human need—not to be parted from all the treasured possessions that are so essential to maintaining our sense of self.

The residents. Are they clean and well groomed? Are they kept occupied, or are most lying in bed or sitting and staring at the wall? Do not expect a camp atmosphere, but expect some residents to be happy and engaged. Approach some of these people, tell them who you are, and ask how they feel about the home. Expect complaints, but also expect to learn a good deal about whether this is a humane place.

The staff. Are they neatly dressed and well groomed? Are they on the floor helping residents? Do they appear to be caring, respectful, and conscientious, answering calls for help without delay? Linger with your eyes and ears open.

The meals and activities. Both are important events in the lives of nursing-home residents. Visit when a meal is being served. Does the food look appetizing, and are there substitutes for the main dish? Do residents who need it get prompt help with eating? Do most eat in the dining room? Visit the activities room. Is it well equipped and staffed? Is a list of activities posted? Do they seem varied, and does the selection include things your loved one would enjoy? Is an effort made to get residents out into the community and bring outsiders in? Is there a volunteer program?

The nursing home should be open to the community, and it should offer residents who are able regular opportunities to leave the grounds. As much as possible, it should also let residents exercise choice, in what they eat, in what they do. As I noted in chapter 3, the ability to make choices enhances not only our psychological well-being but our physical health too.

The medical care. Are there physicians on the staff? Can residents select among them, or are they assigned a doctor? What hospitals are used if your loved one becomes ill? Is this home equipped to provide any needed specialized medical and rehabilitative care?

Health inspection information. Nursing homes are required by law to post the results of the most recent health inspection. However, since inspections occur infrequently and tend to focus on safety violations and the adequacy of the home's physical plant, knowing an institution has passed will not tell much about the quality of care it provides. But information about violations and whether they are being corrected should be used along with your observations as a sign the home is good.

Admissions and cost. If the home seems acceptable, visit the admissions office. Is there a waiting list, and if so, how long? What forms are needed to apply, and how long are applications kept on file? If you are paying privately, what services are included in the basic rate, and what costs are extra? What is the refund policy for leaving prematurely? What is the procedure for applying for Medicaid?

Ideally you will have the luxury of making a fully informed choice. In reality your options are likely to be more limited. If your relative is arriving from the community, the best homes tend to have long waiting lists. Priority is given to patients coming from hospitals. Even if your ideal choice has a wait years long, get on the list. Beds do open up.

If your relative is in the hospital, you may not have time to choose at all. Hospitals used to be paid by the day. According to a new reimbursement method called the DRG system, the hospital is now paid a fixed sum before admission according to the person's "diagnostic related group"—the cost of an estimated "average length of stay" for that condition. This system was devised as an incentive to discourage unnecessarily long hospitalizations. Instead of benefiting economically by keeping patients longer, hospitals now benefit by discharging them sooner, because they collect the same fee regardless of how many days a person stays.

Critics of this system argue that it discriminates against the elderly because, being more frail, they tend to require more time than "average" to recuperate from illness or surgery. Apart from whether this argument has merit, the practical effect of the DRG system is this bottom line: your relative will be pressured to leave the hospital as soon as possible, pushed to accept the first available bed in any area nursing home. But you can forestall this by knowing in advance which homes are acceptable and telling the hospital social worker to call only them. So start your inquiries the minute you think institutional care may be needed—for instance, when your relative enters the hospital.

INVOLVE THE ELDERLY PERSON IN THE PLANS

Once the need becomes obvious, have your relative participate in the decision making and plans—if possible, visiting prospective homes and making the final decision about where to go (when the person is competent to do so). Many families wait until the last minute to break the news, reasoning: "What possible good would the extra months of worry do Mom?" However, consider the pitfalls of waiting: you increase the shock of the move by adding the element of surprise; you add the pain of betrayal. The truth is you have been "putting one over," plotting behind the person's back.

And you rob the elderly person of any chance of control.

Even if your relative has no choice about where to go, breaking the news as soon as possible means choices can be made around the decision. Your mother may be able to arrange to keep her doctor or have her long-standing attendant be there for the first few weeks to make the transition less difficult (it may be psychologically worth the extra expense). She may be able to choose her room or floor, arrange what belongings to take, decide who will come when moving day arrives. Be guided by your knowledge of your relative in following this advice, but also be aware of the research on learned helplessness discussed in chapter 3. In this difficult situation, enhancing control can be lifesaving.

A main fear about nursing homes is the terror of being abandoned, left alone and unloved in an alien place. So as moving day draws near and in the first few weeks, have family and friends make a special effort to rally around. Unless you find that visiting is deeply upsetting, take pains to show your family member you are there. And be as involved as you can for as long as you can.

MONITOR THE CARE IN THE HOME

Research shows that nursing-home residents who have frequent visitors get better treatment. They get more attention from the staff even when visitors are not around.[30] So visiting often will convey to the staff that you are concerned about the care your relative gets. Get to know the nurses and aides on the floor; meet with the doctor and social worker.[31]

If you notice a problem, start out to correct it in a friendly way. Identify the responsible staff member and approach her gently. Give her time to make the change. But if she is unresponsive, do not let sleeping dogs lie. Call the home's administrator, the person who has responsibility for its day-to-day running. If you still get nowhere, then go to the hierarchy's highest level, the home's owner or board of directors.

Or appeal to sources outside the hierarchy. Many homes have a relatives' council or residents' council that meets regularly with the administration to air its concerns. (The presence of either of these organizations is a positive sign the home is responsive to begin with.)

You also can turn to outside advocates. Many communities operate a nursing-home ombudsman program. They employ a person to listen to, investigate, and negotiate solutions to complaints about nursing homes. Your community may have a consumer "watchdog" organization of people interested in nursing-home reform. (Ask the Citizens' Coalition for Nursing Home Reform, based in Washington, D.C., whether a group of this type exists in your area.) These groups not only mediate nursing-home complaints but also offer guidance in selecting a home.

If you stay involved, you are unlikely to need these services. Your relative will be getting good care. And staying close has deeper benefits. You need no longer feel guilty. The person you love has not been put away.

For More Information

CHOOSING AND EVALUATING A DOCTOR (OR SELECTING AN HMO)

American Association of Retired Persons. *More Health for Your Dollar: An Older Person's Guide to HMO's.* Washington, D.C.: AARP, 1983.
This booklet describes HMOs, their advantages and disadvantages, and Medicare coverage. Includes information on how to choose the right HMO.
American Association of Retired Persons. *Health Questions: How to Talk to and Select Physicians, Pharmacists, Dentists, Vision Care Specialists.* Washington, D.C.: AARP, 1985.
This free booklet, published as a public service by the Federal Trade Commission and the AARP, offers information on how to select and evaluate health-care professionals. Write to the AARP, Consumer Affairs Section, Program Department, 1909 K Street N.W., Washington, D.C. 20049, for copies.
County and state medical societies.
Organizations to call for information about the qualifications, training, and affiliation of any prospective doctor.
The Gerontological Society of America, 1411 K Street N.W., Washington, D.C. 20005.
Multidisciplinary group of professionals interested in aging. Pub-

lishes a directory of members. Its Clinical Medicine Section includes some of the doctors interested in geriatrics. Also has information about university-based geriatric centers.

National Institute on Aging, Bethesda, Maryland 20892   (301) 496–1752.
Subdivision of the National Institutes of Health devoted to aging. Conducts research and training as well as funding research and training programs in aging across the country. Will have information about top-quality geriatric centers and programs in your area.

COMMUNITY ALTERNATIVES
TO INSTITUTIONALIZATION

All about Home Care: A Consumer's Guide. Washington, D.C.: National Homecaring Council and Council of Better Business Bureaus, 1983.
Booklet describing home care—when it is needed, how to go about finding services, and how to choose home-care workers wisely. Write to the National Homecaring Council (see below) for copies.

Information Center for Individuals with Disabilities, 20 Providence Street, Boston, Massachusetts 02116   (617) 727–5540.
Helps people with disabilities learn about the appropriate agencies and resources and provides information on promoting a more independent life.

National Council on the Aging, Perspectives on Aging, November/December 1985.
This is the journal of the National Council on the Aging. The whole issue is devoted to day care, describing a variety of programs (write to the NCOA at the address below for copies).

National Homecaring Council, 519 C Street N.E., Washington, D.C. 20002   (202) 547–6586.
Organization devoted to promoting and evaluating home care. Responsible for accrediting agencies and services.

National Institute of Community Based Long-Term Care, National Council on the Aging, 600 Maryland Avenue S.W., Washington, D.C. 20024.
Affiliate of the National Council on the Aging for professionals providing long-term care outside institutions. Represents the range of agencies serving older people at home and in the community.

National Institute on Adult Day Care, National Council on the Aging, 600 Maryland Avenue S.W., West Wing 100, Washington, D.C. 20024 (202) 479-1200.
Division of the National Council on the Aging for professionals working in day-care programs. Disseminates information. Helps people set up day centers. Has an extensive bibliography. Has prepared a national directory of day-care programs.

National League for Nursing, American Public Health Association, 10 Columbus Circle, New York, New York 10019 (212) 582-1022.
Accredits community nursing services such as home health agencies.

Travel Information Service, Moss Rehabilitation Hospital, 12th Street and Tabor Road, Philadelphia, Pennsylvania 19141 (215) 329-5715.
Provides travel information to disabled people and their families for a nominal fee.

MODIFYING THE ENVIRONMENT TO COPE WITH DISABILITIES

LaBuda, D., *The Gadget Book: Ingenious Devices for Easier Living.* Washington, D.C.: AARP Press, 1985.
Lists 350 products and devices to help people deal with arthritis, hearing and vision problems, diminished strength and balance, and other disabilities. Order from your local bookstore or write to AARP Books, Scott, Foresman, 400 South Edward Street, Mount Prospect, Illinois 60056.

Steinfeld, E. *Adaptable Dwellings.* Washington, D.C.: United States Department of Housing and Urban Development, 1979.
Report outlines how devices and design features can be devised to make a home usable for disabled people.

Catalogs of Devices

Abbey Medical: Home Health Care Catalog. Call (714) 962-4477 to find the Abbey location nearest you.

Comfortably Yours: Makes Living Easier. 61 West Hunter Avenue, Maywood, New Jersey 07607 (201) 368-0400.

Enrichments: Catalog for Better Living. Bissell Health Care Companies, P.O. Box 579, Hinsdale, Illinois 60521 (800) 343-9742.

ABOUT NURSING HOMES

American Health Care Association, 1201 L Street N.W., Washington, D.C. 20005   (202) 833-2050.

Federation of state associations serving licensed nursing homes and allied facilities. Members provide long-term care to elderly convalescent and chronically ill people. Publishes consumer guides on nursing-home selection.

American Association of Homes for the Aging, 11292 O Street N.W., Suite 400, Washington, D.C. 20036   (202) 296-5960.

National Association of nonprofit homes and services for the elderly. Also publishes materials on how to choose and evaluate nursing homes.

Flint, M. *A Consumer Guide to Nursing Home Care in New York State*. New York: Friends and Relatives of the Institutionalized Aged, 1987.

Though it applies to nursing homes in New York, this is the best short guide I have come across on how to select and apply for nursing-home care and how to be an effective advocate for a relative should problems arise. Write or call FRIA, 425 East 25th Street, New York, New York 10010   (212) 481-4422 for information about copies.

Mongeau, S., ed. *Directory of Nursing Homes*, 2d ed. Phoenix: Oryx Press, 1984.

Comprehensive state-by-state list of nursing homes, the level of care they provide, certification, admission requirements, special features, activities, and so forth.

National Citizens' Coalition for Nursing Home Reform, 1424 16th Street N.W., Suite L2, Washington, D.C. 20036   (202) 797-0657.

Consumer organization devoted to information and referral, and advocating the rights of nursing-home patients. Publishes information on new federal legislation. Member organizations around the country offer guidance to families in applying for and choosing a nursing home and in advocacy. Perhaps the best single clearinghouse for consumer information on nursing homes.

FINANCING CARE

American Association of Retired Persons, 1909 K Street N.W., Washington, D.C. 20049   (202) 872-4700.

Has information about health-care insurance plus companies offering nursing-home care insurance.

American Association of Retired Persons. *The Prudent Patient: How to Get the Most for Your Health Care Dollar.* Washington, D.C.: AARP, Health Advocacy Services Program Department, 1985.

Booklet offering money-saving tips plus how to get second opinions, what Medicare pays for, HMOs, how to choose a hospital, and so forth.

American Society of Internal Medicine. *Medicare: What It Will and Will Not Pay For.* Washington, D.C.: ASIM, 1981 (updated annually).

Free booklet on what Medicare covers and does not cover. Write to American Society of Internal Medicine, 101 Vermont Avenue N.W., Suite 500, Washington, D.C. 20005, for copies.

Hunt, M. A. "A Common Sense Guide to Health Insurance." *New York Times Magazine,* May 3, 1987.

Excellent article on financing health care and health insurance.

Jehle, F. F. *The Complete and Easy Guide to Social Security and Medicare.* Madison, Conn.: Frasier, 1986.

Book describing in detail what Medicare and Social Security cover.

State Department of Insurance.

Will have information about companies offering long-term care insurance.

(General source for information on the material covered in this chapter: your local office for the aging.)

EPILOGUE

I hope this overview of the psychological research on aging has given you some tools to make the most of your life. In contrast to the bleak stereotype, after age sixty we are emphatically not fated for physical and emotional decrepitude. Decide not to squander these precious years. Enjoy them fully, in the way that fits *your* interests and needs. In these concluding pages are a few suggestions from the many choices open to you.

Furthering Your Education

COLLEGE PROGRAMS

Whether motivated by a pure thirst for learning or by a lifelong dream of getting a degree, increasing numbers of older Americans are pursuing knowledge in its most intense form: they are returning to college. Faced with declining enrollments, schools are embracing this trend, offering tantalizing inducements to older students.

Reduced tuition. More than a thousand colleges across the country either offer reduced fees or waive tuition completely for people over sixty provided there is space in the classes they want to attend. For instance, fee reduction or no charge to elderly students is now standard at many public (state) universities across the country because over half of the state legislatures, who control the state university system, have enacted such laws.

Special programs or courses. According to a 1985 survey by the American Association of Retired Persons, about 120 colleges across the country have modified their offerings to suit the needs of older students, setting up full-blown programs for "retired professionals" or "senior citizens." The most comprehensive ones often include a special curriculum, offer transportation to campus, and provide counseling to help older students adjust to college life.

Some of these programs are completely age segregated. Students take courses only with their own group. Others offer a graduated entry into college life. Students begin by taking special courses and then, when they feel comfortable, begin taking the standard offerings at the school. In yet a third variety students in the program are not segregated at all but are given extensive counseling and help with negotiating college life.

Enrolling in a program of this type offers distinct advantages: being buffered from the bewildering job of registering, choosing courses, and finding your way alone; getting your feet wet academically with people your age; having a built-in chance to make friends. There is often a strong sense of camaraderie among the people who attend these "colleges for retirees."

To find out whether such a program exists in your community, call the admissions office of every nearby college and inquire. Community colleges—because they see their main constituency as adult learners—are likely to be your best bet. State colleges and universities rank second. Special offerings are least likely to be found at private liberal arts colleges. Your local office of the aging or the local chapter of the American Association of Retired Persons should also have information about college programs in your area.

If you want to return to college but cannot find a program of this type, do not be put off. Many college professors are delighted to have older students. Imagine the relief of teaching people who are motivated by a love of learning and whose life experience can add depth to class discussions. By being one of the few gray-haired students on campus, you help enlighten others. Your presence belies the myth that older people are ill and incapable. And in my experience, you are unlikely to be seen as an interloper. Students tend to admire people who after a full working life have the courage and motivation to make a commitment of this magnitude.

You may also be pleasantly surprised about yourself. Studies show that when older people take college courses they tend to get better than average grades, even though many are frightened when they begin—afraid their intellectual abilities won't measure up.

However, having a good experience depends on choosing your college and courses carefully. Don't get in over your head; start out slowly so you can gain confidence. Select high-quality courses and, more important, stimulating professors. Since at this time of life you are liberated from the career consequences of not getting A's, concentrate on having the most intellectually interesting experience you can.

But because you will be such a visible minority in any typical undergraduate institution, be especially sensitive to what the majority wants. You will be seen as an intruder if you talk incessantly or act as if you know it all. If you are auditing courses, understand that your mission is different from that of your fellow students. They are vitally interested in their grades, not just in learning for its own sake. They will not take kindly to your debating fine points with the professor the week before an exam.

LESS INTENSIVE EXPERIENCES

If you want intellectual stimulation but shy away from the intense commitment of college courses, why not enroll in a short-term educational program such as Elderhostel? Elderhostel is a network of over five hundred colleges, universities, and educational institutions that offer special low-cost programs, usually a week long, to people over sixty. There are Elderhostel schools in all fifty states and in Canada, England, and the Scandinavian countries, offering a wide range of liberal arts and science courses. There are no grades, no homework, no exams, and the focus is on making friends and enjoying vacationing as well as learning. Although some people I interviewed had had a disappointing experience with the Elderhostel teachers (or other students), many became addicted to this learning vacation. They loved the mix Elderhostel offers—the chance to travel, meet people, and be intellectually stimulated at the same time.

Or explore the many educational opportunities outside the college campus. Churches, museums, libraries, and YMCAs offer courses and classes in almost every conceivable area. Senior citizens' centers and clubs also offer regular lectures on interesting topics, though their mission is as much social as educational. Nonacademic institutions such as churches or Y's are especially good sources if your educational aims are more creative than academic—if you want to pursue an interest in the arts.

OLDER ARTISTS' GROUPS AND PROGRAMS

Courses in painting or writing or drama are easy to find. However, here too distinct advantages arise from searching out a program specifically for older people. By aligning yourself with an older artists' group, you become a valued commodity. What your group does may be more in demand than if you joined an age-integrated group. If you want to translate what you learn into a second vocation—to exhibit, publish, or perform your work—unexpected doors can open when you capitalize on your creativity and your age.

For instance, at the Jewish Association for Services for the Aged, a philanthropic organization serving older people in the New York area, drama specialists Howard Phlanzer and Susan Miller formed an older adults' theater ensemble by recruiting members from the organization's network of affiliated senior citizens' groups. Some members who passed the audition were in their late eighties. Many had had to abandon a lifelong interest in drama during their working careers. With the help of a historian from Columbia University, the group members wrote a theater piece about their personal experiences—what it was like to be children of immigrants growing up in New York at the turn of the century. Their play aroused the interest of people at the Jewish Museum of the City of New York, and they staged it there to high praise.

Some of the people in this group had attended drama classes at area universities but found they did not offer enough chance to meet people or to perform. Being labeled older gives this group, and the many other artistic groups specifically for people over sixty, special opportunities for public access.

Programs to help, encourage, and train older artists dot the country. To find out what is offered in your community, call or write the state arts council in your state. State arts councils have information about all arts activities including those specifically for people over sixty. And that marvelous general resource—your local office for the aging—should be able to offer you information in this area too.

Finding a Paying Job

As I noted in the chapter on retirement, there is age discrimination in the workplace. But an astonishing one-third to one-quarter of all people go back to work at least for some time after they have formally retired. Most of them take jobs in their previous fields. But some find fulfillment in a completely new occupation or in one they may have been trained for but have hardly worked in at all.

Not all companies practice age discrimination; some even give preference to older workers or retirees. At a recent job fair for older people sponsored by the New York City Department for the Aging, this was evident. The seventy-five exhibitors—banks, retail stores, publishers, and practically every service industry—were spending time and money to seek out people over sixty. Some of our nation's largest, most highly respected corporations have the reputation of looking favorably on hiring older people—Atlantic Richfield, IBM, AT&T, American Express, Burger King, McDonald's, General Electric, Polaroid, and every major insurance company.

This is not to say that finding a satisfying paying job after retirement is easy. It can take a good deal of searching, and it may mean making compromises. Decide which compromises are tolerable and which are unacceptable. Luckily, at this time of life you may have less rigid requirements for a job than you had at twenty-five.

After I retired as vice-president of my company, I went back two days a week as a consultant. I lost my secretary, my clout, and most of my salary, but I gained my freedom. I am surprised at my lack of envy for my colleague in the plush office I used to have. I feel only relief and enjoyment now that the pressure is off.

If, like many retirees who want to return to work, you would prefer a part-time job, the first place to consider is your former company. Ask if you can return as a consultant or work during the busy season when your firm needs extra hands. Being a known quantity, you are likely to have an edge in being hired. Your employer will not have the headache of training you, and you will not have the trauma of adjusting to a new place. (This advice applies only if you were happy there!)

Or consider going into your former field on a smaller scale. If you had an antique shop, could you sell antiques out of a room in your home? Perhaps you could rent part of a warehouse to store your products. If you were an executive secretary, could you free-lance? Call some small neighborhood businesses and tell them you are available to do typing at home. Argue your virtues with their pocketbook in mind: "Wouldn't it be wonderful to hire someone with years of experience who could also save your company money by working out of her home?"

If neither returning to your old company nor becoming self-employed is feasible, you must muster the courage to tackle a job search. Job specialists at the New York City Department for the Aging advise concentrating your efforts on these two fronts: combing the want ads and telling everyone you are looking for work. In their experience, these avenues are more productive than visiting employment agencies. Another approach they find surprisingly effective is to call places "cold." If you want a job as a legal secretary, look up lawyers in the Yellow Pages. Start with Aardvark and Jones and work your way down. Try to bypass personnel departments—ask for Mr. Aardvark himself. (The worst that can happen is they tell you he died in 1945.) Expect rebuffs, and forge ahead. Spend time. "Finding a job is a job itself" applies doubly today.

Use a schedule to organize yourself. Consider yourself self-employed in the occupation "job searcher." Schedule your day in the same way you would if you were genuinely self-employed: "From 9:00 to 11:00 A.M. each day, I'll look through the want ads and call prospects. I must visit five agencies within the next three weeks." "There are four people I think may be helpful. My deadline for calling them is April 1."

Use a similar strategy when you "network," or ask people you know for help. Instead of saying, "Do me a favor; I need work desperately," and then waiting by the phone, give the person a deadline: "I would appreciate your telling Mr. Jones about me. I'll call you back on Friday to find out what he says." If people know you will be calling them again by a certain date, they are more likely to follow through.

Search intelligently, taking your "maturity" into account. Concentrate on industries and companies that are age friendly. Your state labor department may have a "mature worker," unit with these listings. Or find out if your area has a private agency that specializes in placing older employees. Your local office for the aging may operate an employment service, offering workshops in job-finding skills as well as training and placement services. (Unfortunately, these services are often restricted to low-income elderly.) Your local library, churches, or YMCA may also offer job counseling. Community colleges are another good source. Their career counseling centers are sometimes open to anyone in the community, not just students.

If you have sought out an employer who is looking for a "mature worker," the age issue is not there. Generally, however, you will not be interviewing for a position that is preselected in this way. How can you deal with your emotions and put a positive cast on your age during an interview?

DEALING WITH YOUR AGE IN A JOB INTERVIEW

Some older job applicants are so sure their age is a liability that they enter interviews with an air of defensiveness that almost ensures failure. If this scenario might fit you, make a special effort to prevent it. Prime yourself by listing your positive qualities. Study what your prospective employer needs and be able to spell out exactly why you as a mature person (or just as a person) are best for the job. You might rehearse answers to these age-related concerns: Hiring you may cost more. You will be less satisfied with the salary a younger person would accept. Benefits will have to be paid out earlier. The company's health-insurance premiums may go up. The investment of time in training you will not be made up by years of productive work. Teaching you will also be more difficult. Not only are older people more set in their ways, they are likely to be emotionally incapable of taking instruction from a younger boss.

If these doubts come up directly, be ready to counter them gracefully. You are enthusiastic, healthy, and prepared to stay on the job. You just had a medical checkup, and your doctor

says you have the stamina of a person of thirty-five. The salary
is not everything (if true); you want to work as much for self-
fulfillment as for a wage. You cannot wait to learn those new
techniques. "It will be so nice to be in an atmosphere where I
can learn from the younger people around." Because no employer wants to feel inferior to an employee—and many people
do have qualms about being "boss" to someone their parents'
age—this last point may be particularly important to get
across. Subtly reassure the interviewer that you will not be a
threat.

Here are some reasons, adapted from the AARP pamphlet
Working Options: How to Plan Your Job Search, why older
people make good employees.

Job loyalty. On average, older workers stay on a job three
times as long.

Less absenteeism. Older workers are more reliable and
punctual.

Good skills. Experience and judgment are their forte; they
often have better writing, spelling, and math abilities too.

Conscientiousness. They work harder and take more pride
in the job.

Grace under pressure. Because of their greater maturity,
older workers are less likely to get hysterical or fly off the handle in a crisis.

At the same time as you seriously address any anxieties your
age evokes, it also may help to inject some humor. For instance, here is an anecdote that a senatorial candidate of sixty-
eight often told when the age issue was brought up: "When I
mentioned to my ninety-seven-year-old mother that my age is
a problem in this race, she said, 'Nonsense son, I think you're
old enough to run.'"

In tackling the job search, be encouraged by this fact. In a
front page article in July 1986, the *Wall Street Journal* reported
that today more candidates in their sixties, seventies, and
even eighties are running for public office than ever before.
Rather than deemphasizing their age, many of these older office seekers are now accentuating it, arguing that their additional years of life experience make them better qualified to

govern. The strategy is working; many or most have won. If people in this appearance-oriented occupation can transform being older from a liability into an asset, so can you!

Volunteer Work

Although getting a paycheck is satisfying, there are heartaches involved in searching for a paying job. If you are among the many retirees who want to work for psychological, not monetary rewards, volunteering may be a more fulfilling route.

As a volunteer you can try your hand in a totally new field; you have more freedom to select your hours; you do not have to waste precious months in a frustrating job search. You also have a satisfying intangible reward—the admiration of others and of yourself.

Volunteer work is not "less important." It can involve the ultimate in responsibility. Consider, for instance, the volunteer position member of the board of directors or board of trustees. It is hard to argue that overseeing the running of universities or hospitals is unimportant simply because these people are not being paid.

Older people who volunteer are a special group. They tend to be healthier and better educated than the average person their age. They donate their time for reasons as different as doing good for their fellowman and getting out of the house. A common reason is to tie up loose ends. Volunteering is tailor-made for satisfying unfulfilled dreams.

I always wanted to be a doctor, but I never got the chance. After I retired from the post office, I began volunteering in a hospital emergency room. I'm a kind of patient representative and jack-of-all-trades, doing anything short of performing surgery. When I'm in my white coat, I feel as if I really had gone to medical school. The patients call me doctor, and I sometimes forget to correct them. I'm having more fun than I've had in years!

Older people are the backbone of volunteer programs in practically every community organization—schools, hospitals, churches, nursing homes, museums, zoos. Some volunteers make more than a full-time commitment, such as joining the Peace Corps; others lick envelopes a few hours a month.

If this route to self-fulfillment appeals to you, be systematic.

Analyze what you want to get out of being a volunteer. Think about your priorities and search for the setting that best fits your needs. For instance, if you want to work with children but also are volunteering in order to meet people and get out of the house, choose a job in a school over tutoring individual students in your home. Carefully consider your sensitivities. Would you find working in an institution for the retarded too depressing, or would you relish it as a challenging experience?

Check out potential jobs carefully. Unfortunately, placements may vary greatly in the quality of the experience they offer volunteers. For jobs where you have responsibility for other people—working in a school or a hospital, visiting disabled people who can't get out of the house—expect some training. High-quality programs offer orientation sessions and ongoing supervision once you are in the field. They are also selective, not accepting everyone who applies. You may be asked to provide references or a résumé. Since these positions can involve a good deal of responsibility for people's welfare, these requirements are reasonable. Be wary if you are accepted automatically for any demanding volunteer job or thrown into a sensitive new situation unprepared.

Before accepting a position, do some interviewing yourself. Question volunteers already at the organization. In some places volunteers are resented by the paid employees, restricted to unsatisfying tasks, or as just mentioned, cut adrift to flounder alone. A frank discussion with current volunteers about problems they are having with help you avoid a placement of this type.

Another way of minimizing the risk of a bad experience is to get your placement through a volunteer bureau. No agency would keep sending its volunteers to settings where they were mistreated. Working through an agency is also advisable for learning about your alternatives and solidifying your interests.

Often counseling is offered to help people focus on exactly what they want to do. An agency will also monitor problems that arise and offer further counseling and another placement if things do not work out.

Take your job seriously. Once on the job, make the same commitment you would if you were receiving a paycheck. Be reliable; complete your assignments; respect the confidences of clients you serve. Volunteer work is far from "optional." If it were, there would be no point in considering it a valuable way to spend your time.

While many agencies place volunteers of any age, four sponsored by the federal government are just for people sixty and over: the Retired Senior Volunteer Program (RSVP), the Service Corps of Retired Executives (SCORE), and the Foster Grandparent and Senior Companion programs. There also are many excellent local volunteer agencies for older people throughout the country.

RSVP is by far the largest older adult volunteer program, with over a quarter of a million participants serving on nearly seven hundred projects in all fifty states. With its far-ranging roster of placements and its national reputation, it makes sense to look into RSVP first, particularly if you are not sure where you want to work and are volunteering in part to meet people your own age. Participants in RSVP get together for various functions such as parties and lectures. In fact this organization combines some of the social features of a club with those of an agency.

The other three national older persons' volunteer programs are much more limited in scope. SCORE, sponsored by the Small Business Administration, is specifically for retired businessmen who want to use their skills in helping others. People in this program offer small businesses assistance and guidance in accounting, finance, advertising, marketing, taxation, and other aspects of management.

The famous Foster Grandparent Program and the newer, less known Senior Companion Program are only for low-income people. Both ask for a substantial part-time commitment. In return, volunteers get transportation to their placements, meals while on the job, intensive training and supervision, and a small weekly stipend.

Foster grandparents serve as caring grandparents to emotionally disturbed and physically or mentally handicapped children. They provide two hours of individual attention to each of two children daily, time no one else is able to offer. Foster grandparents usually work in institutions for the handicapped or in schools. However, as is true in a Texas project where foster grandparents work with abused and neglected infants and also teach good child-rearing techniques, they sometimes donate their time at the child's home.

Senior companions serve the opposite end of the age spectrum, physically and mentally impaired older adults. During a usually twenty-hour week, a senior companion visits several homebound clients, either to talk—perhaps offering the only human contact the disabled person may get—or to provide concrete help. Senior companions read, shop, and take walks with their clients. They may help them fill out Medicaid forms or apply for food stamps. One of the unique aspects of this program is the ongoing close relationship that develops between clients and volunteers. As with any good volunteer experience, both the giver and the receiver benefit. In the words of one senior companion whose visits have kept an older client from having to enter a nursing home: "I'm happy for the first time since the children left home and I broke up housekeeping. Pauline's been as good for me as I am for her."

Just as volunteering has given this woman a sense of purpose, you should demand the same from any of the doors that swing open by virtue of your being a "mature" adult. Do not waste these priceless years succumbing to outmoded stereotypes about what age sixty or eighty is supposed to mean. Make this your time to flower!

For More Information

GOING BACK TO COLLEGE OR TAKING COURSES

American Association of Retired Persons. *Learning Opportunities for Older People.* Washington, D.C.: Institute of Lifetime Learning, AARP, 1985.
Booklet describing the general types of institutions offering programs and information about additional resources related to adult

education. For copies, write to the Institute of Lifetime Learning (address above).

The American Association of Retired Persons. *Tuition Policies for Older Adults.* Washington, D.C.: Institute of Lifetime Learning, AARP, 1985.
This national directory compiled by the AARP lists by state most of the colleges and universities offering older people reduced tuition or special programs, or both.

Elderhostel, 100 Boylston Street, Boston, Massachusetts 02116 (617) 426–8056.
The largest, best-established vacation/learning service for people over sixty. Write or call for information and a catalog.

Institute of Lifetime Learning, American Association of Retired Persons, 1909 K Street N. W., Washington, D.C. 20049.
This is the educational enrichment arm of the AARP, promoting opportunities for older people to go back to college and prepare for second careers and also publishing materials related to lifetime learning.

Ventura-Merkel, C. *Education for Older Adults: A Catalogue of Program Profiles.* Washington, D.C.: National Council on the Aging, 1983.
Describes sixteen educational programs for older people operated by colleges, unions, libraries, and offices of the aging. Illustrates the range of opportunities that exist.

Weinstock, R. *The Graying of the Campus.* New York: Educational Facilities Laboratory, 1978.
Aimed at college administrators but also relevant to older people considering going back to college. This book discusses who returns to college after retirement, the needs of this group, and what qualities make special college programs for older people work.

OLDER ARTISTS' GROUPS

Cahil, P. *Arts, the Humanities, and Older Americans: A Catalogue of Program Profiles.* Washington, D.C.: National Council on the Aging, 1981.
Describes three dozen programs in the humanities for and by older people. Although some may no longer be operating, this booklet illustrates the diversity that exists.

Center for Arts and the Aging, National Council on the Aging, 600

Maryland Avenue S.W., West Wing 100, Washington, D.C. 20024 (202) 479–1200.

Program of the National Council on the Aging devoted to promoting the arts and humanities. Publishes material relating to the arts and aging (see below); encourages older artists' groups. Operates a gallery that exhibits the work of older artists from across the nation.

McCutcheon, P. B., and C. S. Wolf. *A Resource Guide to People, Places, and Programs in the Arts and Aging.* Washington, D.C.: National Council on the Aging, 1984.

A directory of programs in the arts and aging by state. Also offers short descriptions of the more than fifty programs listed.

FINDING NEW EMPLOYMENT

Brochures, Books, and Newsletters

The American Association of Retired Persons. *Second Career Opportunities for Older Persons.* Washington, D.C.: AARP, 1985.

American Association of Retired Persons. *Working Options: How to Plan Your Job Search, Your Work Life.* Washington, D.C.: AARP, 1985.

Brochures relevant to choosing a second career and finding a job. Write to AARP, 1909 K Street N.W., Washington, D.C. 20049 for copies.

Crawley, B., and J. Dancy. *Mature/Older Job Seeker's Guide.* Washington, D.C.: National Council on the Aging, 1984.

Danna, J. *It's Never Too Late to Start Over.* Briarwood, N.Y.: Palomino Press, 1983.

Books offering advice on how to look for a job and market yourself as an older worker.

Older Worker News, National Association of Older Worker Employment Services, National Council on the Aging, Washington, D.C. Newsletter of a professional interest group whose focus is improving employment opportunities for older adults. Offers information on national employment policies and news about innovative programs for older workers and employment opportunities.

Working Age, AARP Worker Equity Department, Washington, D.C. Bimonthly newsletter sent free to organizations interested in issues of employment for older people. Also provides information about legislation and programs affecting older workers.

Employment Agencies and Services

Displaced Homemakers Network, 1411 K Street N.W., Suite 930, Washington, D.C. 20005.
Offers help to homemakers in preparing for employment.

Forty-Plus Clubs, 1718 P Street N.W., Washington, D.C. 20036.
Nonprofit peer-run employment service with branches in major cities for out-of-work executives over age forty. (People must have previously earned more than $30,000 a year to quality.) Members offer one another support in finding a job and developing good job-searching strategies.

Mature Temps, 1114 Avenue of the Americas, New York, New York 10036.
Agency with branches in major cities specializing in placing older temporary office workers.

(Also consult your local office for the aging, library, YMCA, or community college for help.)

VOLUNTEERING

ACTION, the National Volunteer Agency, 806 Connecticut Avenue N.W., Washington, D.C. 20525 (800) 424–8867 or (202) 634–9424).
This is the federal agency that administers RSVP, the Foster Grandparent and Senior Companion programs, the Peace Corps, and more. Write for information about these programs; look in your White Pages for regional offices.

AARP Talent Bank, Volunteer Bank, 1909 K Street N.W., Washington, D.C. 20049.
Identifies volunteers and refers them to agencies nationwide. Publishes informational guides about volunteering.

American Association of Retired Persons. *To Serve Not Be Served: A Guide for Volunteers.* Washington, D.C.: AARP, 1985.
Offers information on volunteering—what will be expected of you, and your rights, Write to AARP, Program Department for free copies.

RSVP, the Retired Senior Volunteer Program. Washington, D.C.: ACTION, 1987.
Booklet describing the operation and activities of this largest volunteer program for older adults. Write to ACTION for copies.

SCORE, Small Business Administration, 1129 20th Street N.W.,

Suite 410, Washington, D.C. 20036   (800) 368-5855.
Volunteer program for retired business executives. Call or write
the address above for information about local chapters, or check
your local phone book under Small Business Administration and
inquire.

(Also, call your local office of the aging. Look in your Yellow Pages
under volunteer agencies.)

N O T E S

Chapter 1: The Body

1. E. B. Palmore, "Trends in the Health of the Aged," *Gerontologist* 26 (1986): 298–302.
2. G. A. Kaplan, "Aging, Health, and Behavior: Evidence from the Alameda County Study," paper presented at the ninety-fourth annual meeting of the American Psychological Association, Washington, D.C., August 1986.
3. E. Shanus, "Old Parents and Middle Aged Children: The Four and Five Generation Family," *Journal of Geriatric Psychiatry* 17 (1984): 7–19.
4. C. Longino, "The Oldest Americans: Their Demographic, Socioeconomic, Relational and Environmental Characteristics," paper presented at the thirty-ninth annual meeting of the Gerontological Society of America, Chicago, November 1986.
5. N. W. Shock, R. C. Greulich, R. Andres, D. Arenberg, P. Costa, E. G. Lakatta, and J. D. Tobin, *Normal Human Aging: The Baltimore Longitudinal Study of Aging*, National Institutes of Health publication 84-2450 (Rockville, Md.: National Institute on Aging, 1984).
6. Unless otherwise noted, the information in this section comes from S. Whitbourne, *The Aging Body: Physiological Changes and Psychological Consequences* (New York: Springer-Verlag, 1985); J. K. Belsky, *The Psychology of Aging: Theory, Research, and Practice* (Monterey, Calif.: Brooks/Cole, 1984); and these National Institute on Aging Age Pages: *Aging and Your Eyes; Hearing and the Elderly; Digestive Dos and Don'ts; Constipation*.
7. See, for instance, S. Schiffman and M. Pasternack, "Decreased Discrimination of Food Odors in the Elderly," *Journal of Gerontology* 34 (1979): 73–79.
8. University of Chicago psychologist Robert Kahn was the first to use this evocative phrase, one he felt fit the situation of a large number of patients in nursing homes.
9. S. E. Levkoff, P. D. Cleary, and T. Wetle, "Differences in the Appraisal of Health between Aged and Middle Aged Adults," *Journal of Gerontology* 42 (1987): 114–20.
10. P. Lamy, "Patterns of Prescribing and Drug Use," in *The Aging Process: Therapeutic Implications*, ed. R. N. Butler (New York: Raven Press, 1985).
11. From *Safe Use of Medicines by Older People*, a National Institute on Aging Age Page.
12. K. Rost and D. Roter, "Predictors of Recall of Medication Regi-

mens and Recommendations for Lifestyle Change in Elderly Patients,"
Gerontologist 27 (1987): 510–15.

13. Many of these suggestions are from R. West, *Memory Fitness over Forty* (Gainesville, Fla.: Triad, 1985).

Chapter 2: The Mind

1. J. Rodin and E. Langer, "Aging Labels: The Decline of Control and the Fall of Self-Esteem," *Journal of Social Issues* 36 (1980): 12–29.

2. For instance, researchers have shown that even doctors, nurses, mental health workers, and people who work in nursing homes tend to make this misattribution.

3. R. West, L. K. Boatwright, and R. Schleser, "The Link between Memory Performance, Self-Assessment, and Affective Status," *Experimental Aging Research* 10 (1984): 197–200.

4. While not all studies show a link between memory complaints and depression, many do. This research was recently reviewed by psychologist George Neiderehe in "Depression and Memory Dysfunction in the Aged," paper presented at the thirty-ninth annual meeting of the Gerontological Society of America, Chicago, November 1986.

5. K. W. Schaie and G. Labouvie-Vief, "Generational versus Ontogenetic Components of Change in Adult Cognitive Behavior: A Fourteen Year Cross-Sequential Study," *Developmental Psychology* 10 (1974): 305–20.

6. G. Labouvie-Vief, "Modes of Knowing and Life-Span Cognition," and F. Blanchard-Fields, "Self, Other, and Progressions in Adult Cognition," papers presented at the ninety-fourth annual meeting of the American Psychological Association, Washington, D.C., August 1986.

7. J. L. Horn, "Organization of Data on Life-Span Development of Human Abilities," in *Lifespan Developmental Psychology: Research and Theory*, ed. L. R. Goulet and P. B. Baltes (New York: Academic Press, 1970).

8. K. Gribbon, K. W. Schaie, and I. A. Parham, "Complexity of Lifestyle and Maintenance of Intellectual Abilities," *Journal of Social Issues* 36 (1980): 47–61.

9. A. Fengler, "Productivity and Representation: The Elderly Legislator in State Politics," paper presented at the twenty-ninth annual meeting of the Gerontological Society of America, New York, November 1976.

10. S. J. Buell and P. D. Coleman, "Dendritic Growth in the Aged Human Brain and Failure of Growth in Senile Dementia," *Science* 206 (1979): 854–56.

11. The behavioral counterpart to this is that in advanced old age *crystallized* intelligence does markedly fall off, an unfortunate reality underlined most recently by neuropsychiatrist Lissy Jarvik in "Aging of the Brain: How Can We Prevent It?" a paper presented at the fortieth

annual meeting of the Gerontological Society of America, Washington, D.C., November 1987.

12. J. A. Hopson, "A Love Affair with the Brain: *PT* Conversation with Marian Diamond," *Psychology Today* 18 (1984): 62.

13. P. Brook, G. Degun, and M. Mather, "Reality Orientation, a Therapy for Psychogeriatric Patients: A Controlled Study," *British Journal of Psychiatry* 127 (1975): 42–45.

14. R. Larson, J. Zuzanek, and R. Mannell, "Being Alone versus Being with People: Disengagement in the Daily Experience of Older Adults," *Journal of Gerontology* 40 (1985): 375–81.

15. L. Harris and associates, *Aging in the Eighties: America in Transition* (Washington, D.C.: National Council on the Aging, 1981).

16. For instance, for more than a quarter-century gerontologists have known that even asymptomatic chronic disease can lower IQ. See J. Botwinick and J. E. Birren, "Mental Abilities and Psychomotor Responses in Healthy Aged Men," in *Human Aging: A Biological and Behavioral Study*, ed. J. E. Birren, R. N. Butler, S. W. Greenhouse, L. Sokoloff, and M. R. Yarrow (Washington, D.C.: United States Public Health Service, 1963).

17. United States Department of Health and Human Services, Public Health Service, *Medicine for the Layman: The Brain in Aging and Dementia*, NIH publication 83-2625 (Bethesda, Md.: National Institutes of Health, 1983).

18. The following description is taken from F. I. M. Craik, "Age Differences in Human Memory," in *Handbook of the Psychology of Aging*, ed. J. E. Birren and K. W. Schaie (New York: Van Nostrand-Reinhold, 1977).

19. G. A. Sperling, "A Model for Visual Memory Tasks," *Human Factors* 5 (1963): 19–31.

20. I. M. Hulicka and J. L. Grossman, "Age Group Comparisons for the Use of Mediators in Paired Associate Learning," *Journal of Gerontology* 22 (1967): 46–51.

21. R. E. Canestrari, "Paced and Self-Paced Learning in Young and Elderly Adults," *Journal of Gerontology* 18 (1963): 165–68.

22. These two techniques are adapted from B. Furst, *Stop Forgetting* (New York: Doubleday, 1972).

23. This strategy is adapted from R. West, *Memory Fitness over Forty* (Gainesville, Fla.: Triad Press, 1985).

Chapter 3: Personality

1. C. G. Jung, "The Stages of Life," trans. R. F. C. Hull, in *The Portable Jung*, ed. J. Campbell (New York: Viking, 1971).

2. B. L. Neugarten, "The Awareness of Middle Age," in *Middle Age*, ed. R. Owen (London: British Broadcasting Corporation, 1967).

3. B. L. Neugarten and associates, *Personality in Middle and Late Life* (New York: Atherton, 1964).

4. For instance, see L. M. Gambria, "Sex Differences in Day-Dreaming and Related Mental Activity from the Late Teens to the Early Nineties," *International Journal of Aging and Human Development* 10 (1979–80): 1–34; M. F. Lowenthal, M. Thurnher, and D. Chiriboga, *Four Stages of Life* (San Francisco: Jossey-Bass, 1975); and the chapter on retirement below (chap. 6).

5. Paul Costa, the preeminent advocate of personality consistency (see the next section), is one of the most vocal critics.

6. D. L. Gutmann, "Male Parenthood and Mastery Style: A Druse Example," paper presented at the International Congress of Gerontology, July 1985, New York.

7. K. L. Cooper and D. L. Gutmann, "Gender Identity and Ego Mastery Style in Middle-Aged, Pre- and Post-Empty Nest Women," *Gerontologist* 27 (1987): 347–52.

8. See, for instance, M. M. Weismann, J. K. Myers, G. L. Tischler, C. E. Holtzer III, P. J. Leaf, H. Orvascel, and J. A. Brody, "Psychiatric Disorders (DSM III) and Cognitive Impairment among the Elderly in a U.S. Urban Community," *Acta Psychiatra Scandinavica* 71 (1985): 366–79; M. C. Feinson and P. A. Thoits, "The Distribution of Distress among Elders," *Journal of Gerontology* 41 (1986): 225–33; D. S. Butt and M. Beiser, "Successful Aging: A Theme for International Psychology," *Psychology and Aging* 2 (1987): 87–94.

9. L. F. Jarvik and D. Russell, "Anxiety, Aging and the Third Emergency Reaction," *Journal of Gerontology* 34 (1979): 197–200.

10. R. R. McCrea, "Age Differences in the Use of Coping Mechanisms," *Journal of Gerontology*, 37 (1982): 454–60.

11. Although not all studies, by far, show that older people handle stress in a more mature way, this encouraging finding is not an isolated one. For another recent study showing this, see J. C. Iron and F. Blanchard-Fields, "A Cross-Sectional Comparison of Adaptive Coping in Adulthood," *Journal of Gerontology* 42 (1987): 502–4.

12. N. Shock, R. C. Greulich, R. Andres, and D. Arenberg, *Normal Human Aging: The Baltimore Longitudinal Study of Aging*, NIH publication 84-2450 (Rockville, Md.: National Institute on Aging, 1987).

13. K. Ell, M. Mantell, and M. Hamovich, "Adaptation to Cancer among Different Age Cohorts," paper presented at the thirty-ninth annual meeting of the Gerontological Society of America, Chicago, November 1986.

14. For instance, see R. R. McCrea and P. T. Costa, *Emerging Lives, Enduring Dispositions: Personality in Adulthood* (Boston: Little, Brown, 1984).

15. P. T. Costa, A. B. Zonderman, R. R. McCrea, J. Cornoni-Huntley, B. Z. Locke, and H. E. Barbano, "Longitudinal Analyses of Psychological Well-Being in a National Sample: Stability of Mean Levels," *Journal of Gerontology* 42 (1987): 50–55.

16. H. Maas and J. A. Kuypers, *From Thirty to Seventy: A Forty Year Study of Adult Lifestyles and Personality* (San Francisco: Jossey-Bass, 1974).

17. The radically different idea that we change a good deal during adulthood and that shifting life situations are probably what cause this change was also the conclusion of a recent study tracing the lives of some of the children of Maas and Kuypers's subjects. See N. Haan, R. Millsap, and E. Hartka, "As Time Goes By: Change and Stability in Personality over Fifty Years," *Psychology and Aging* 1 (1986): 220–32.

18. D. M. Ogilvie, "Life Satisfaction and Identity Structure in Late Middle-Aged Men and Women," *Psychology and Aging* 2 (1987): 217–24.

19. M. F. Lowenthal, P. L. Berkman, and associates, *Aging and Mental Disorder in San Francisco* (San Francisco: Jossey-Bass, 1967).

20. G. Kaplan, "Aging, Health, and Behavior: Evidence from the Alameda County Study," paper presented at the ninety-fourth annual meeting of the American Psychological Association, Washington, D.C., August 1986.

21. For just one recent example, see D. M. Gibson, "Interaction and Well-Being in Old Age: Is It Quantity or Quality That Counts?" *International Journal of Aging and Human Development* 24 (1986–87): 29–33.

22. As reported in J. Rodin, "Aging and Health: Effects of the Sense of Control," *Science* 233 (1986): 1271–76.

23. J. Rodin, "Physiological Mediators of Health and Behavior: Relationships in Aging," paper presented at the ninety-fourth annual meeting of the American Psychological Association, Washington, D.C., August 1986.

24. Much of the information in this section is adapted from G. L. Klerman, "Problems in the Diagnosis of Depression in the Elderly," in *Depression and Aging: Causes, Care, and Consequences*, ed. L. Breslau and M. R. Haug (New York: Springer, 1983).

25. D. Gallagher, L. Thompson, and J. S. Breckenridge, "Maintenance of Gains versus Relapse Following Brief Psychotherapy for Depression," paper presented at the ninety-fourth annual meeting of the American Psychological Association, Washington, D.C., August 1986.

Chapter 4: Love, Marriage, and Sex

1. L. Ade-Ridder and T. H. Brubaker, "The Quality of Long-Term Marriages," in *Family Relationships in Later Life*, ed. T. H. Brubaker (Beverly Hills, Calif.: Sage, 1983).

2. R. C. Atchley and S. Miller, "Types of Elderly Couples," in *Family Relationships in Later Life*, ed. T. H. Brubaker (Beverly Hills, Calif.: Sage, 1983).

3. M. Fitting, P. Rabins, M. J. Lucas, and J. Eastham, "Caregivers for

Dementia Patients: A Comparison of Husbands and Wives," *Gerontologist* 26 (1986): 248–52.

4. C. L. Johnson, "The Impact of Illness on Late-Life Marriages," *Journal of Marriage and the Family* 47 (1985): 165–72.

5. For instance, see C. E. Depner and B. Ingersol-Dayton, "Conjugal Social Support: Patterns in Later Life," *Journal of Gerontology* 40 (1985): 761–66.

6. J. Cuber and P. Haroff, *Sex and Significant Americans* (New York: Appleton-Century-Crofts, 1965).

7. C. L. Cole, "Marital Quality in Later Life," in *Independent Aging: Family and Social Systems Perspectives*, ed. W. H. Quinn and G. A. Hughston (Rockville, Md.: Aspen, 1984).

8. E. L. Kelly and J. J. Conley, "Personality and Compatibility: A Prospective Analysis of Marital Stability and Marital Satisfaction," *Journal of Personality and Social Psychology* 52 (1987): 27–40.

9. K. Bulcroft and M. O'Connor-Rodin, "Never Too Late," *Psychology Today* 20 (1986): 66–69.

10. H. G. Pieper, L. Petkovsek, and M. East, "Marriage among the Elderly," paper presented at the thirty-ninth annual meeting of the Gerontological Society of America, Chicago, November 1986.

11. E. M. Brecher and the editors of Consumer Reports Books, *Love, Sex, and Aging* (Boston: Little, Brown, 1984).

12. In addition to journal articles, the Duke and Baltimore findings on sexuality are in these books: E. Palmore, ed., *Normal Aging*, vols. 1 and 2 (Durham, N.C.: Duke University Press, 1970, 1974); and N. W. Schock and associates, *Normal Human Aging: The Baltimore Longitudinal Study of Aging* (Rockville, Md.: National Institute on Aging, 1984).

13. W. H. Masters and V. E. Johnson, *Human Sexual Response* (Boston: Little, Brown, 1966).

14. Brecher, *Love, Sex, and Aging*, 34–35.

15. In all three studies—Duke, Baltimore, and Consumers Union—people who reported the highest levels of sexual interest also reported the highest levels of interest and activity in their youth.

16. Most of the information in these sections is taken from articles in *Sex over Forty* from 1982 to 1986.

17. Brecher, *Love, Sex, and Aging*, 369.

18. Ibid.

19. See A. Bloch, J. Maeder, and J. Haissly, "Sexual Problems after Myocardial Infarction," *American Heart Journal* 90 (1975): 536–37.

20. *Sex over Forty.*

21. Masters and Johnson, *Human Sexual Response.*

22. C. V. Christenson and J. H. Gagnon, "Sexual Behavior in a Group of Older Women," *Journal of Gerontology* 20 (1965): 351–56.

23. Much of the information in this section is from Jane Brody's "Personal Health" column in the *New York Times*, February 25, 1987. Brody was reporting on the findings of a consensus conference on osteoporosis held at the National Insitute on Aging in early 1987.

24. Brecher, *Love, Sex, and Aging.*

Chapter 5: The Generations

1. E. Shanas, "Old People and Their Families: The New Pioneers," *Journal of Marriage and the Family* 42 (1980): 9–18.

2. E. M. Brody, "Parent Care as a Normative Family Stress," *Gerontologist* 25 (1985): 19–28.

3. E. Shanus, "The Family as a Social Support System in Old Age," *Gerontologist* 19 (1979): 169–74.

4. See E. Litwak and C. F. Longino, "Migration Patterns among the Elderly: A Developmental Perspective," *Gerontologist* 27 (1987): 266–72; and C. F. Longino, "Migration Winners and Losers," *American Demographics* 6 (1984): 27–29.

5. Brody, "Parent Care."

6. Ibid.

7. W. H. Jarrett, "Caregiving within Kinship Systems: Is Affection Really Necessary?" *Gerontologist* 25 (1985): 5–10.

8. R. Aisenberg and J. Treas, "The Family in Late Life: Psychosocial and Demographic Considerations," in *Handbook of the Psychology of Aging*, 2d ed., ed. J. E. Birren and K. W. Schaie (New York: Van Nostrand-Reinhold, 1985).

9. I. O. Okraku, "Age and Attitudes towards Multi-generational Residence, 1973–1983," *Journal of Gerontology* 42 (1987): 280–87.

10. T. Kausar and A. Wistar, "Living Arrangements of Older Women: The Ethnic Dimension," *Journal of Marriage and the Family* 46 (1984): 301–10.

11. See B. J. Cohler and H. V. Grunebaum, *Mothers, Grandmothers, and Daughters: Personality and Childcare in Three-Generation Families* (New York: Wiley, 1981); and G. O. Hagestad, "Continuity and Connectedness," in *Grandparenthood*, ed. V. L. Bengston and J. F. Robertson (Beverly Hills, Calif.: Sage, 1985).

12. J. A. Kuypers and V. L. Bengston, "Toward Competence in the Older Family," in *Family Relations in Late Life*, ed. T. H. Brubaker (Beverly Hills, Calif.: Sage, 1983).

13. C. Johnson, "Grandparenting Options in Divorcing Families: An Anthropological Perspective," in *Grandparenthood*, ed. V. L. Bengston and J. F. Robertson (Beverly Hills, Calif.: Sage, 1985).

14. For instance, see G. R. Lee and E. Ellithorpe, "Intergenerational Exchange and Subjective Well Being among the Elderly," *Journal of Marriage and the Family* 44 (1982): 217–24; and T. Quinn, "Personal and Family Adjustment in Later Life," *Journal of Marriage and the Family* 45 (1983): 57–73.

15. D. Callahan, "What Do Children Owe Their Elderly Parents?" *Hastings Center Report* 15 (1985): 32–37.

16. Ibid.

17. Callahan reproduced this quotation from Irving Kristol's review of Ben Wattenberg's *The Good News is Bad News* (New York: Simon and Schuster, 1984), in *New Republic*, October 29, 36.

18. These statistics are from the United States Senate, Special Com-

mittee on Aging, *Aging America: Trends and Projections*, 1985–86 ed. (Washington, D.C.: United States Senate, Special Committee on Aging, 1984).

19. C. Johnson and D. Catalano, "A Longitudinal Study of Family Supports to Impaired Elderly," *Gerontologist* 23 (1983): 612–18.

20. L. R. Fisher, "Elderly Parents and the Caregiving Role: An Asymmetrical Transition," in *Social Bonds in Later Life*, ed. W. Peterson and J. Quadagno (Beverly Hills, Calif.: Sage, 1985).

21. S. H. Zarit, K. Reever, and J. Bach-Peterson, "Relatives of the Impaired Elderly: Correlates of Feelings of Burden," *Gerontologist* 20 (1980): 649–55.

22. S. Zarit, N. Orr, and J. Zarit, *The Hidden Victims of Alzheimer's Disease: Families under Stress* (New York: New York University Press, 1985).

23. E. P. Stoller, "Exchange Patterns in the Informal Support Networks of the Elderly: The Impact of Reciprocity on Morale," *Journal of Marriage and the Family* 47 (1985): 335–42.

24. L. E. Troll, "Grandparents: The Family Watchdogs," in *Family Relationships in Later Life*, ed. T. H. Brubaker (Beverly Hills, Calif.: Sage, 1983).

25. Hagestad, "Continuity and Connectedness."

26. Johnson, "Grandparenting Options in Divorcing Families."

27. B. Neugarten and K. K. Weinstein, "The Changing American Grandparent," *Journal of Marriage and the Family* 26 (1984): 199–204.

28. A. Cherlin and F. Furstenberg, "Styles and Strategies of Grandparenting," in *Grandparenthood*, ed. V. L. Bengston and J. F. Robertson (Beverly Hills, Calif.: Sage, 1985).

29. Johnson, "Grandparenting Options in Divorcing Families."

30. Hagestad, "Continuity and Connectedness."

31. C. L. Johnson and B. M. Barer, "Marital Instability and the Changing Kinship Networks of Grandparents," *Gerontologist* 27 (1987): 330–35.

Chapter 6: Retirement

1. The statistics in this section are from United States Senate, Special Committee on Aging, *Aging America: Trends and Projections*, 1985–86 ed. (Washington, D.C.: United States Senate, Special Committee on Aging, 1984).

2. Ibid.

3. For a similar set of conclusions see R. F. Boaz, "The 1983 Amendments to the Social Security Act: Will They Delay Retirement? A Summary of the Evidence," *Gerontologist* 27 (1987): 151–55.

4. E. Palmore, B. Birchett, G. G. Fillenbaum, L. K. George, and L. M. Wallman, *Retirement: Causes and Consequences* (New York: Springer, 1985).

5. United States Senate, *Aging America.*

6. See G. G. Fillenbaum, "On the Relation between Attitude to Work and Attitude to Retirement," *Journal of Gerontology* 26 (1971): 244–48; and F. D. Glamser, "Determinants of a Positive Attitude towards Retirement," *Journal of Gerontology* 31 (1976): 104–7.

7. L. Evans, D. Ekerdt, and R. Bosse, "Proximity to Retirement and Anticipatory Involvement: Findings from the Normative Aging Study," *Journal of Gerontology* 40 (1985): 368–74.

8. See the discussion of David Gutmann's research in chapter 3.

9. M. Lowenthal, M. Thurnher, D. Chiriboga, and associates, *Four Stages of Life: A Comparative Study of Men and Women Facing Transitions* (San Francisco: Jossey-Bass, 1975).

10. D. J. Ekerdt, "The Busy Ethic: Moral Continuity between Work and Retirement," *Gerontologist* 26 (1986): 239–44.

11. Palmore et al., *Retirement.*

12. A. Foner and K. Schwab, *Aging and Retirement* (Monterey, Calif.: Brooks/Cole, 1981).

13. H. L. Sheppard, "Work and Retirement," in *Handbook of Aging and the Social Sciences,* ed. E. Shanas and R. H. Binstock (New York: Van Nostrand-Reinhold, 1976).

14. United States Senate, *Aging America.*

15. P. Robinson, S. Coberly, and C. Paul, "Work and Retirement," in *Handbook of Aging and the Social Sciences,* 2d ed., ed. R. H. Binstock and E. Shanas (New York: Van Nostrand-Reinhold, 1986).

16. Sheppard, "Work and Retirement."

17. United States Senate, *Aging America.*

18. Palmore et al., *Retirement.*

19. United States Senate, *Aging America.*

20. Palmore et al., *Retirement;* G. Streib and C. J. Schneider, *Retirement in American Society: Impact and Process* (Ithaca, N.Y.: Cornell University Press, 1971).

21. United States Senate, *Aging America.*

22. Palmore et al., *Retirement;* Streib and Schneider, *Retirement in American Society.*

23. L. Harris and associates, *Aging in the Eighties: America in Transition* (Washington, D.C.: National Council on the Aging, 1981).

24. D. S. Butt and M. Beiser, "Successful Aging: A Theme for International Psychology," *Psychology and Aging* 2 (1987): 87–94.

25. United States Senate, *Aging America.*

26. W. Usui, T. Keil, and K. R. Durig, "Socioeconomic Comparisons and Life Satisfaction of Elderly Adults," *Journal of Gerontology* 40 (1985): 110–14.

27. J. M. Strate and S. J. Dubnoff, "How Much Income Is Enough? Measuring the Income Adequacy of Retired Persons Using a Survey Based Approach," *Journal of Gerontology* 41 (1986): 393–400.

28. Palmore et al., *Retirement.*

29. Streib and Schneider, *Retirement in American Society.*

30. S. Reichard, F. Livson, and P. Peterson, *Aging and Personality* (New York: Wiley, 1962).

31. D. J. Ekerdt, R. Bosse, and S. Levkoff, "An Empirical Test for Phases of Retirement: Findings from the Normative Aging Study," *Journal of Gerontology* 40 (1985): 95–101.

32. Palmore et al., *Retirement.*

Chapter 7: Widowhood

1. C. M. Parkes, *Bereavement: Studies of Grief in Adult Life* (New York: International Universities Press, 1972), 93.

2. The statistics in this section are from United States Senate, Special Committee on Aging, *Aging America: Trends and Projections*, 1985–86 ed. (Washington, D.C.: United States Senate, Special Committee on Aging, 1984); and P. Silverman, *Helping Women Cope with Grief* (Beverly Hills, Calif.: Sage, 1981).

3. Ibid.

4. J. Treas and A. Van Hilst, "Marriage and Remarriage Rates among Older Americans," *Gerontologist* 16 (1976): 132–36.

5. W. Cleveland and D. Gianturco, "Remarriage Probability after Widowhood: A Retrospective Method," *Journal of Gerontology* 31 (1976): 99–103.

6. H. Z. Lopata, *Widowhood in an American City* (Cambridge, Mass.: Schenkman, 1973).

7. T. Rando, *Grief, Dying, and Death: Clinical Interventions for Caregivers* (Champaign, Ill.: Research Press, 1984).

8. K. J. Helsling, M. Szklo, and G. W. Comstock, "Factors Associated with Mortality after Widowhood," *American Journal of Public Health* 71 (1981): 802–9.

9. See M. C. Feinson, "Aging Widows and Widowers: Are There Mental Health Differences?" *International Journal of Aging and Human Development* 23 (1986): 241–50; and D. A. Lund, M. S. Caserta, and M. F. Dimond, "Gender Differences through Two Years of Bereavement among the Elderly," *Gerontologist* 26 (1986): 314–20.

10. N. Krause, "Social Support, Stress, and Well Being among Older Adults," *Journal of Gerontology* 41 (1986): 512–19.

11. This research was recently discussed by D. L. Morgan in "Social Networks and Adjustment to Widowhood," paper presented at the fortieth annual meeting of the Gerontological Society of America, Washington, D.C., November 1987.

12. Lopata, *Widowhood in an American City.*

13. E. Lindemann, "Symptomatology and Management of Acute Grief," *American Journal of Psychiatry* 101 (1944): 141–48.

14. Rando, *Grief, Dying, and Death.*

15. J. W. Worden, *Grief Counseling and Grief Therapy* (New York: Springer, 1982).

16. Rando, *Grief, Dying, and Death;* Worden, *Grief Counseling and Grief Therapy.*

17. Rando, *Grief, Dying, and Death.*

18. Ibid.

19. Ibid.

20. From K. Lorenz, *On Aggression* (London: Methuen, 1963), as quoted in Worden, *Grief Counseling,* 8–9.

21. J. Bowlby, *Loss* (New York: Basic Books, 1980).

22. J. N. Breckenridge, D. Gallagher, L. W. Thompson, and J. Peterson, "Characteristic Depressive Symptoms of Bereaved Elders," *Journal of Gerontology* 41 (1986): 163–68.

23. Rando, *Grief, Dying, and Death.*

24. C. M. Parkes and R. S. Weiss, *Recovery from Bereavement* (New York: Basic Books, 1983).

25. Rando, *Grief, Dying, and Death.*

26. Ibid.

Chapter 8: Living Arrangements and Changing Residence

1. The statistics in this section are from United States Senate, Special Committee on Aging, *Aging America: Trends and Projections,* 1985–86 ed. (Washington, D.C.: United States Senate, Special Committee on Aging, 1984).

2. See C. Longino, "Migration Winners and Losers," *American Demographics* 6 (1984): 27–29; and C. B. Flynn, C. F. Longino, R. F. Wiseman, and J. C. Biggar, "The Redistribution of America's Older Population: Major National Migration Patterns for Three Census Decades, 1960–1980," *Gerontologist* 25 (1985): 292–96.

3. E. Litwak and C. F. Longino, "Migration Patterns among the Elderly: A Developmental Perspective," *Gerontologist* 27 (1987): 266–72.

4. United States Senate, *Aging America.*

5. American Association for Retired Persons, *DATA GRAM: Housing Satisfaction in Older Americans* (Washington, D.C.: AARP, 1984).

6. M. Weinberger, J. C. Darnell, B. L. Martz, S. Hiner, P. O'Neill, and W. M. Tierney, "The Effects of Positive and Negative Life Changes on the Self-Reported Health Status of Elderly Adults," *Journal of Gerontology* 41 (1986): 114–20.

7. S. Sherwood, J. Glassman, C. Sherwood, and J. N. Morris, "Preinstitutional Factors as Predictors of Adjustment to a Long-Term Care Facility," *International Journal of Aging and Human Development* 5 (1974): 95–105.

8. B. F. Turner, S. S. Tobin, and M. A. Lieberman, "Personality Traits as Predictors of Institutional Adaptation among the Aged," *Journal of Gerontology* 27 (1972): 681–86.

9. F. M. Carp, "Short-Term and Long-Term Prediction of Adjustment to a New Environment," *Journal of Gerontology* 29 (1974): 444–53.

10. F. M. Carp, "Relevance of Personality Traits to Adjustment in Group Living Situations," *Journal of Gerontology* 40 (1985): 544–51.

11. K. Moos and S. Lemke, "Specialized Living Environments for Older People," in *Handbook of the Psychology of Aging*, 2d ed., ed. J. E. Birren and K. W. Schaie (New York: Van Nostrand-Reinhold, 1985).

12. Most of this information is from L. Hubbard and T. Beck, eds., *Housing Options for Older Americans* (Washington, D.C.: AARP, 1984).

13. The Greens at Leisure World is at 14901 Pennfield Circle, Silver Spring, Maryland 20906 (301) 598–2500.

14. Goodwin House is at 4800 Fillmore Avenue, Alexandria, Virginia 22311 (703) 578–1000.

15. Otterbein Home is at 585 North State Street, Route 7, Lebanon, Ohio 45036 (513) 932–2020.

16. A. J. La Greca, G. F. Streib, and W. E. Folts, "Retirement Communities and Their Life Stages," *Journal of Gerontology* 40 (1985): 211–18.

17. L. G. Branch, "Continuing Care Retirement Communities: Self-Insuring for Long-Term Care," *Gerontologist* 27 (1987): 4–8.

18. "Life-Care Communities: Protecting the Residents," seminar at the thirty-sixth annual meeting of the National Council on the Aging, Washington, D.C., April 1986.

19. F. E. Netting and C. C. Wilson, "Current Legislation concerning Life-Care and Continuing Care Contracts," *Gerontologist* 27 (1987): 645–51.

20. American Association of Homes for the Aging, *The Continuing Care Retirement Community: A Guidebook for Consumers* (Washington, D.C.: American Association of Homes for the Aging, 1984).

21. Hubbard and Beck, *Housing Options for Older Americans*.

22. K. Kenny and B. Belling, "Home Equity Conversion: A Counseling Model," *Gerontologist* 27 (1987): 9–12.

23. Hubbard and Beck, *Housing Options for Older Americans*.

24. Ibid.

25. Ibid.

Chapter 9: Dementia

1. B. Chenoweth and B. Spenser, "Dementia: The Experience of Family Caregivers," *Gerontologist* 26 (1987): 266–72.

2. Gurland gave this description at a symposium on Alzheimer's disease held at Columbia University in June 1985.

3. S. Zarit, N. Orr, and J. Zarit, *The Hidden Victims of Alzheimer's Disease: Families under Stress* (New York: New York University Press, 1985); see also B. Reisberg, *Brain Failure: An Introduction to Current Concepts of Senility* (New York: Free Press, 1981).

4. S. Zarit, P. A. Todd, and N. Zarit, "Subjective Burden of Husbands and Wives as Caregivers: A Longitudinal Study," *Gerontologist* 26 (1986): 260–66.

5. S. Borson, L. Teri, A. Kyak, and R. Montgomery, "Behavioral Syndromes in Alzheimer's Disease: Relationship to Cognitive and Functional Impairments," paper delivered at the thirty-ninth annual meeting of the Gerontological Society of America, Chicago, November 1986.

6. Zarit, Orr, and Zarit, *Hidden Victims of Alzheimer's Disease*.

7. G. Wolff-Klein, F. Silverstone, A. Levy, V. Termatto, M. Brod, and C. Foley, "Are Alzheimer Patients Healthier?" paper presented at the thirty-ninth annual meeting of the Gerontological Society of America, Chicago, November 1986.

8. Zarit, Orr, and Zarit, *Hidden Victims of Alzheimer's Disease*.

9. Ibid.

10. Ibid.; V. C. Hashinski, N. A. Lassen, and J. Marshal, "Multi-infarct Dementia," *Lancet* 2 (1974): 207–9.

11. Zarit, Orr, and Zarit, *Hidden Victims of Alzheimer's Disease*.

12. Ibid.; M. Roth, "Evidence on the Possible Heterogeneity of Alzheimer's Disease and Its Bearing on Future Inquiries into Etiology and Treatment," in *The Aging Process: Therapeutic Implications*, ed. R. N. Butler and A. G. Bearn (New York: Raven, 1985).

13. H. M. Fillit, E. Kemeny, V. Luine, M. Wekskler, and J. B. Zabriskie, "Antivascular Antibodies in the Sera of Patients with Senile Dementia of the Alzheimer's Type," *Journal of Gerontology* 42 (1987): 180–84.

14. D. Barnes, "Defect in Alzheimer's is on Chromosome 21," *Science* 234 (1987): 846–47.

15. Ibid.

16. G. Mckhann, D. Drachman, M. Folstein, R. Katzman, D. Price, and E. M. Stadlan, "Clinical Diagnosis of Alzheimer's Disease: Report of the NINCDS-ADRDA Work Group Under the Auspices of the Department of Health and Human Services Task Force on Alzheimer's Disease," *Neurology* 34 (1984): 939–44.

17. B. Habot and L. S. Libow, "The Interrelationship of Mental and Physical Status and Its Assessment in the Older Adult: Mind-Body Interaction," in *Handbook of Mental Health and Aging*, ed. J. E. Birren and R. B. Sloane (Englewood Cliffs, N.J.: Prentice-Hall, 1980).

18. R. I. Block, M. DeVoe, B. Stanley, M. Stanley, and N. Pomara, "Memory Performance in Individuals with Primary Degenerative Dementia: Its Similarity to Diazepam-Induced Impairments," *Experimental Aging Research* 11 (1985): 151–55.

19. R. B. Sloane, "Organic Brain Syndrome," in *Handbook of Mental Health and Aging*, ed. J. E. Birren and R. B. Sloane (Englewood-Cliffs, N.J.: Prentice-Hall, 1980).

20. Chenoweth and Spenser, "Dementia."

21. Zarit, Orr, and Zarit, *Hidden Victims of Alzheimer's Disease*; Mckhann et al., "Clinical Diagnosis of Alzheimer's Disease."

22. E. B. Larson, B. V. Reifler, S. M. Sumi, C. G. Canfield, and N. M. Chinn, "Diagnostic Evaluation of 200 Elderly Outpatients with Suspected Dementia," *Journal of Gerontology* 40 (1985): 536–43.

23. Roth, "Evidence on the Possible Heterogeneity of Alzheimer's Disease."

24. Larson et al., "Diagnostic Evaluation of Elderly Outpatients."

25. Zarit, Orr, and Zarit, *Hidden Victims of Alzheimer's Disease.*

26. Ibid., 165.

27. L. K. George and L. P. Gwyther, "Caregiver Well-Being: A Multidimensional Examination of Family Caregivers of Demented Adults," *Gerontologist* 26 (1986): 253–58.

28. Zarit, Orr, and Zarit, *Hidden Victims of Alzheimer's Disease;* Zarit, Todd, and Zarit, "Subjective Burden of Husbands and Wives as Caregivers"; L. P. Gwyther and L. K. George, "Caregivers for Dementia Patients: Complex Determinants of Well-Being and Burden," *Gerontologist* 26 (1986): 245–47.

29. Zarit, Orr, and Zarit, *Hidden Victims of Alzheimer's Disease.*

30. C. L. Johnson, "Dyadic Family Relationships and Family Supports: An Analysis of the Family Caregiver," *Gerontologist* 23 (1983): 377–83.

31. J. Kahan, B. Kemp, F. Staples, and K. Brummel-Smith, "Decreasing the Burden in Families Caring for a Relative with a Dementing Illness: A Controlled Study, *Journal of the American Geriatrics Society* 33 (1985): 664–70.

Chapter 10: Disability and Health Care

1. The statistics in this section are from United States Senate, Special Committee on Aging, *Aging America: Trends and Projections*, 1985–86 ed. (Washington, D.C.: United States Senate, Special Committee on Aging, 1984).

2. M. E. Williams and J. C. Hornberger, "A Quantitative Method of Identifying Older Persons at Risk for Increasing Long Term Care Services," *Journal of Chronic Diseases* 37 (1984): 705–11.

3. For an analysis of the variety of predictors of nursing-home placement, see D. L. Wingard, D. Williams Jones, and R. M. Kaplan, "Institutional Care Utilization by the Elderly," *Gerontologist* 27 (1987): 156–63.

4. T. F. Williams, "Geriatrics: The Fruition of the Clinician Reconsidered," *Gerontologist* 26 (1986): 345–49.

5. R. L. Kane, D. H. Solomon, J. C. Beck, E. Keeler, and R. A. Kane, *Geriatrics in the United States: Manpower Projections and Training Considerations* (Lexington, Mass.: Heath, 1981).

6. Ibid.

7. G. Adams, *Essentials of Geriatric Medicine* (New York: Oxford University Press, 1977).

8. M. G. Greene, S. Hoffman, R. Charon, and R. Adelman, "Psychosocial Concerns in the Medical Encounter: A Comparison of the Interactions of Doctors with Their Young and Old Patients," *Gerontologist* 27 (1987): 164–68.

9. M. R. Haug, ed., *Elderly Patients and Their Doctors* (New York: Springer, 1981).

10. T. N. Chirikos and G. Nestel, "Longitudinal Analysis of Functional Disabilities in Older Men," *Journal of Gerontology* 40 (1985): 426–33.

11. P. H. Liem, R. Chernoff, and W. J. Carter, "Geriatric Rehabilitation Unit: A Three Year Outcome Evaluation," *Journal of Gerontology* 41 (1986): 44–50.

12. United States Senate, *Aging America.*

13. Some of the information in this section is adapted from American Association of Retired Persons, *Healthy Questions: How to Talk to and Select Physicians, Pharmacists, Dentists, Vision Care Specialists* (Washington, D.C.: AARP, 1985).

14. The information here is adapted from American Association of Retired Persons, *More Health for Your Dollar: An Older Person's Guide to HMO's* (Washington, D.C.: AARP, 1983).

15. As reported in M. A. Hunt, "A Common Sense Guide to Health Insurance," *New York Times Magazine,* May 3, 1987.

16. Ibid.

17. Psychologist Andrew Dibner invented this widely available program, Lifeline Systems, Inc., Watertown, Massachusetts 02172.

18. J. H. Hodgson and J. L. Quinn, "The Impact of the Triage Health Care Delivery System upon Client Morale, Independent Living, and the Cost of Care," *Gerontologist* 20 (1980): 364–71.

19. K. L. Braun and C. L. Rose, "Geriatric Patient Outcomes and Costs in Three Settings: Nursing Home, Foster Family, and Own Home," *Journal of the American Geriatrics Society* 35 (1987): 387–97.

20. United States Senate, *Aging America.*

21. Hunt, "Common Sense Guide to Health Insurance."

22. J. M. Weiner, D. A. Ehrenworth, and D. A. Spense, "Private Long-Term Care Insurance: Cost, Coverage, and Restrictions," *Gerontologist* 27 (1987): 487–93.

23. Hunt, "Common Sense Guide to Health Insurance."

24. The information in this section is from *All about Home Care: A Consumer's Guide* (New York: National Homecaring Council and Council of Better Business Bureaus, 1983).

25. K. Smith and V. L. Bengston, "Positive Consequences of Institutionalization: Solidarity between Parents and Their Middle Aged Children," *Gerontologist* 19 (1979): 438–47.

26. J. Retsinas and P. Garrity, "Going Home: Analysis of Nursing Home Discharges," *Gerontologist* 26 (1986): 431–36.

27. J. I. Kosberg, "Making Institutions Accountable: Research and Policy Issues," *Gerontologist* 14 (1974): 510–16.

28. S. Lemke and R. H. Moos, "Quality of Residential Settings for Elderly Adults," *Journal of Gerontology* 41 (1986): 268–76.

29. This information is from M. L. Flint, *A Consumer Guide to Nursing Home Care in New York State* (New York: Friends and Relatives of the Institutionalized Aged, 1982).

30. L. E. Gottesman and N. C. Bournstam, "Why Nursing Homes Do What They Do," *Gerontologist* 14 (1974): 501–6.

31. Flint, *Consumer Guide to Nursing Home Care.*

INDEX

Accusations, insulting, 239

Acetylcholine, 232

Activity, 43, 71; mental, 44, 49

Activity levels, changes in, 77

Addison's disease, 227; and depression, 77

Adjustment, after death of spouse, 172

Adult children: as advisers, 120; and aging parent relationships, 122; and parental advice, 121–22; and parental attention, 122

Advice giving: between generations, 119–20; problems of, 120; topics of, 120–21; to widowed persons, 181

Age discrimination, 150, 151, 285

Age limit, maximum, 4

Aging: advancement of, 10; affects of, 12–13; and athletics, 12–13; differences in, 9, 10, 24; and IQ, 35, 38; and memory, 35; normal, 10

Agitation, 241

Alameda County (Calif.), 7, 73; home-equity plans in, 209

Albert, Prince, 171

Alcohol: and impotence, 101, 104; use of, 21

Alcoholics Anonymous, 84

Alexandria, Va., Goodwin House, 197

Aluminum, and Alzheimer's disease, 224

Alzheimer's disease, 40, 44, 77, 127, 218, 219, 222, 223–26, 240, 241, 271; causes of, 224–25; diagnosis of, 226; and Down's syndrome, 225; false diagnosis of, 226; and memory, 47, 49; progress rate, 221; risks of getting, 225–26; tests for, 229–31;

treatment of, 231–33. *See also* Dementia

Alzheimer's Disease and Related Disorders Association, 230, 232–33, 239, 241, 267; newsletter of, 232–33

Amended Age Discrimination in Employment Act, 146

American Association of Homes for the Aging checklist, 204

American Association of Retired Persons (AARP), 190, 281, 282, 288; Widowed Persons' Service, 184

American Express, 285

American Heart Association, 267

American Psychological Association, 7, 36, 40, 76, 80

Amyloid, 225

Anger, 127, 128; as a symptom of bereavement, 174, 175, 176

Angina, medications for, 107

Anonymity, loss of, 199

Antibiotics, 6

Anxiety, 48, 200, 201; medication for, and impotence, 104; and memory, 54, 56; and retirement, 148–49; and tranquilizers, 233

Apartments, accessory, 209–10

Appetite changes, 23, 77

Arizona, as a retirement destination, 188, 189

Arteriosclerosis, 7, 44; and impotence, 104. *See also* Dementia, multi-infarct

Arthritis, 7, 246, 247

Arthritis Foundation, 267

Artist's groups, 284

Assimilation, and widowhood, 169

Association, in memory, 52

AT&T, 285

Atchley, Robert, 90, 93, 157